Nurse–Client Communication: A Life Span Approach

Deborah Antai-Otong, MS, APRN, BC, FAAN
Program Manager, Employee Support Program
Organizational Consultant
Veterans Affairs
North Texas Health Care System
Dallas, Texas

JONES AND BARTLETT PUBLISHERS
Sudbury, Massachusetts
BOSTON   TORONTO   LONDON   SINGAPORE

World Headquarters
Jones and Bartlett Publishers
40 Tall Pine Drive
Sudbury, MA 01776
978-443-5000
info@jbpub.com
www.jbpub.com

Jones and Bartlett Publishers Canada
6339 Ormindale Way
Mississauga, Ontario L5V 1J2
CANADA

Jones and Bartlett Publishers International
Barb House, Barb Mews
London W6 7PA
UK

Jones and Bartlett's books and products are available through most bookstores and online booksellers. To contact Jones and Bartlett Publishers directly, call 800-832-0034, fax 978-443-8000, or visit our website, www.jbpub.com.

Substantial discounts on bulk quantities of Jones and Bartlett's publications are available to corporations, professional associations, and other qualified organizations. For details and specific discount information, contact the special sales department at Jones and Bartlett via the above contact information or send an email to specialsales@jbpub.com.

Library of Congress Cataloging-in-Publication Data
Antai-Otong, Deborah.
  Nurse-client communication : a life span approach / Deborah Antai-Otong.
      p. ; cm.
  Includes bibliographical references.
  ISBN-13: 978-0-7637-3588-3 (pbk.)
  ISBN-10: 0-7637-3588-4
  1. Nurse and patient. 2. Communication in nursing.
  [DNLM: 1. Nurse-Patient Relations. 2. Communication. WY 87 A535n 2006] I. Title.
  RT86.3.A58 2006
  610.73—dc22

                                                                                      2006002655
6048

Production Credits
Acquisitions Editor: Kevin Sullivan
Associate Editor: Amy Sibley
Production Director: Amy Rose
Associate Production Editor: Kate Hennessy
Marketing Manager: Emily Ekle
Composition: Auburn Associates, Inc.
Manufacturing and Inventory Coordinator: Amy Bacus
Cover Design: Kristin E. Ohlin
Printing and Binding: Malloy, Inc.
Cover Printing: Malloy, Inc

Printed in the United States of America
10 09 08 07 06   10 9 8 7 6 5 4 3 2

Dedication

This book is dedicated to my best friend and husband, Okon, whose continual support, encouragement, and patience inspired me to undertake this great venture. A special dedication is also extended to my grandparents, Walter and Onie, whose warmth and love continue to inspire me.

Contents

Preface ix

**Chapter One Perspectives and Principles of Therapeutic
Communication** 1

   Learning Objectives 1
   Key Terms. 2
   Introduction 3
   Communication Theories 5
   Factors and Trends Associated with Communication 9
   Modes of Communication. 27
   Legal and Ethical Considerations 35
   Summary 41
   Suggestions for Clinical and Experiential Activities 41
   End-of-Chapter Questions and Answers 43
   Research Study 1–1 44

Chapter Two Therapeutic Communication Techniques 53

   Learning Objectives 53
   Key Terms. 54
   Introduction 55
   Therapeutic Communication Techniques 57
   Critical Thinking Questions 62
   Life Span Considerations 84
   Critical Thinking Question 90
   Chapter Summary. 91
   Suggestions for Clinical and Experiential Activities 91
   End-of-Chapter Questions and Answers 92
   Research Study 2–1 94

**Chapter Three Nurse–Client Interactions:
Strengthening Care Partnerships** 99

   Learning Objectives 99

Key Terms. 99
Introduction 99
The Nurse–Client Relationship 103
The Impact of Technologies on Interpersonal Relationships 108
Self-Awareness and Personal Development. 111
Life Span Considerations 113
Collaborative Relationships 119
Ethical and Legal Considerations 122
End-of-Life Communication 124
Critical Thinking Question 135
Summary 140
Suggestions for Clinical and Experiential Activities 141
End-of-Chapter Questions and Answers 142
Research Study 3–1 143
Research Study 3–2 144

Chapter Four Cultural Aspects of Communication Partnerships **153**
Learning Objectives 153
Key Terms. 154
Introduction 154
Changing Demographics. 157
Health Care Disparities. 159
Communication Considerations of Cultural Competence 162
Culture and Communication across the Life Span 172
Critical Thinking Question 176
Summary 183
Suggestions for Clinical and Experiential Activities 184
End-of-Chapter Questions and Answers 186
Research Study 4–1 187

Chapter Five Professional Development: Leading through Effective
Communication **195**
Learning Objectives 195
Key Terms. 196
Introduction 196
What Constitutes an Effective Leader?. 199
Systems Thinking 205
Professional Assertiveness. 206

Shared Decision Making 207
Conflict Management 213
Critical Thinking Question 214
Negotiation Skills 215
Team-Building Skills 217
Public Speaking Skills 225
Self-Renewal: The Forgotten Leadership Competence 227
Summary 229
Suggestions for Clinical and Experiential Activities 230
End-of-Chapter Questions and Answers 230
Research Study 5–1 232
Research Study 5–2 233

Index **239**

Preface

It is a privilege to write *Nurse–Client Communication: A Life Span Approach* during the revolution of telecommunication, which has had a great impact on how people communicate. Communication is fundamental to survival and is transmitted through various means including language, words, symbols, rituals, customs, dress, body language, and information technologies. From the prenatal period through death, communication enables humans to interact and share ideas, attitudes, beliefs, express joy, pain, sadness, and various feelings with others. Communication is grounded in human behaviors within various social contexts; hence, it is difficult to fathom interpersonal transactions without it. Consequently, communication is fundamental to all nursing and interpersonal relationships.

Today's nurses are challenged to communicate within various social contexts and healthcare arenas. Advances in information technologies, changes in societal demographics, and a greater emphasis on interdisciplinary teams to deliver quality and individualized health care necessitate astute listening and interpersonal skills. Daily encounters with clients, families, and clinicians require communication skills that foster helping and healing environments to optimize clinical outcomes. An aging society, a rise in chronic illnesses and health disparities, and greater emphasis on the provision of evidence-based care require nurses to establish partnerships with clients, families, clinicians, and stakeholders to ensure appropriate resource allocation and parity in healthcare services.

This book has been written in part to help students and also novice and experienced nurses strengthen their interpersonal and communication skills. Basic and complex communication concepts, such as active listening, self-awareness, the nurse–client relationship, negotiation, conflict management, and team building are also discussed as venues to help the client and family navigate complex health care systems and optimize health care. Self-awareness and professional and leadership skills are crucial communication tools that must be developed and used as the foundation of quality nurse–client relationships. Prepared with confidence, astute communication, and interpersonal skills, the nurse can establish shared and participatory decision making with the client, family, and colleagues. Collectively, this approach can ensure that assessment information is accurately interpreted and communicated and that that information is then used to guide the treatment planning and facilitate positive outcomes across the life span.

The following discussion provides a synopsis of each chapter. Strategies discussed throughout the book offer students and nurses opportunities to use self-awareness to learn about themselves and how they relate to others. More importantly, nurse–client encounters can enhance their communication skills and confidence to facilitate optimal functional status in clients and families across the life span.

Chapter One focuses on developing basic communication skills. Communication theories, modes of communication, and factors that influence communication introduce the reader to the basis of communication patterns. It also provides a litany of therapeutic communication techniques to establish rapport, trust, and convey empathy and understanding—the basis of quality therapeutic nurse–client relationships. Societal trends, including the explosion of information technologies and biological, psychosocial, and cultural factors are also discussed. Life span issues provide the reader with the evolution of communication, the impact of early relationships with parents and caregivers as the basis of adult behavior and communication patterns. Ethical and legal considerations that impact communication are also detailed in this chapter.

Chapter Two focuses primarily on therapeutic techniques that strengthen nurse–client encounters. Nurse–client dialogues are used throughout the chapter. Dialogues provide examples of various communication techniques, such as active listening, conflict resolution, paraphrasing, and distinguish between assertive, passive, and aggressive communication. Critical thinking questions are used to stimulate decision making. Barriers to active listening as well as essential characteristics that promote effective communication are also delineated. Overall, this chapter provides techniques that facilitate self-awareness and strengthen interpersonal relationships with clients, families, and healthcare providers.

Chapter Three describes the significance of the nurse–client relationship partnerships within a rapidly changing healthcare arena to preserve client integrity and respect, facilitate optimal levels of functioning, and create healthy work environments. Shared decision making, healthcare partnerships, and collaborative approaches are discussed to expand and optimize the needs of clients across the life span. Self-awareness and personal development are also discussed as part of how the nurse relates to others. Effective communication and quality nurse–client relationships are used to address difficult decisions, such as palliative care or end-of-life issues.

Chapter Four explicates the cultural aspects of communication. Greater emphasis is placed on providing holistic and client-centered care based on client values, beliefs, health practices, and wishes. It also describes the importance of self-awareness when caring for clients whose beliefs, values, and culture differ from that of the nurse. Collectively, this chapter raises awareness concerning the uniqueness of *all* clients and the need to develop nurse–client relationships that optimize the client's needs.

Chapter Five is unique because of its emphasis on personal and professional development. It stresses the importance of leadership and self-renewal in creating environments in which the student, novice, or experienced nurse can act professionally and personally. It emphasizes the role of the nurse in helping the client navigate complex healthcare systems using quality communication and interpersonal skills. Leadership, systems thinking, team building, negotiation, shared decision making, conflict resolution, and other important communication skills are addressed as an integral aspect of professional and personal development. Public speaking skills and self-renewal finalize this chapter.

As nurses we have a responsibility to use each encounter as a venue to create quality and effective interactions with clients and our colleagues. We must extend this approach to nurse colleagues to optimize our contributions to healthy work environments and to advance the needs of clients and ourselves. I believe that we treat people the way we feel about ourselves. Feeling good and respecting ourselves enables us to nurture these qualities in our clients, nurse colleagues, families, and team members. Self-awareness is critical to this process. It enables each nurse to transcend socialization issues, which have historically impeded nurses from nurturing each other and expanding personal and professional development. This book offers suggestions and guidance in developing self-awareness and confidence to optimize our communication and interpersonal skills in various social contexts.

Chapter One

Perspectives and Principles of Therapeutic Communication

LEARNING OBJECTIVES

Upon completion of this chapter, the reader should be able to:

- Define communication and its significance to nursing

- Discuss communication theories and their relevance to nurse–client interactions

- Analyze major factors and trends associated with communication

- Describe communication across the life span and how it applies to nursing

- Analyze major components of effective communication

KEY TERMS

Aphasia—The loss of the ability to comprehend or generate language.

Attachment—A lasting affectional tie or emotional bond, initially between the infant and primary caregivers; it involves seeking closeness to one or more caregivers to feel safe and secure and as a means of understanding the world.

Attachment theory—Based on the classic works of Bowlby and Ainsworth that describe attachment or bonding as an adaptive evolutionary and biological process of eliciting and governing physical closeness between an infant and primary caregiver or parent. The integrity of these early child–parent interactions is believed to influence future relationships, trust, and reliance on others.

Body language—Nonverbal communication or transmission of a message by way of physical gestures or behaviors.

Broca's area—Located in the temporal region of the brain, it is involved in the production of speech; it processes information received from Wernicke's area into a complex and synchronized pattern for vocalization and projects the pattern through a speech articulation region to the motor cortex.

Communication—The act or reciprocal process of imparting or interchanging thoughts, attitudes, emotions, opinions, or information by speech, writing, or signs.

Emotional competence—An individual's ideas, thoughts, motivations, and adeptness for establishing interpersonal relationships.

Empathy—The experience of sharing the feelings, thoughts, and ideas of another. It is a process in which the nurse "puts him- or herself in the client's shoes" without the experience becoming his or her own. It allows for emotional connectedness and understanding without becoming the nurse's experience. It is the opposite of sympathy.

Language—A complex process and mechanism used to communicate.

Personal space—One's comfort zone or space or space surrounding a person's body in interpersonal relationships. It is often influenced by cultural factors and trust.

Professional boundaries—Rules that define who participates in the interpersonal relationship and how they interact; they define the nature of interactions and roles in relationships, and protect the separateness of the nurse–client relationship.

Rapport—A harmonious, empathetic, and mutually respectful relationship between the nurse and client.

Self-awareness—Personal insight or recognition of one's attitudes, biases, values, beliefs, and ideas and the impact they have on relationships with others.

Speech—The motor act of communicating through articulation and verbal expression.

Sympathy—Identification with the client's situation, feelings, and thoughts; difficulty removing oneself from a client's experience. It is the opposite of empathy.

Therapeutic communication—A healing or curative interaction between individuals.

Transactions—Patterns of interactions or communication between people.

Wernicke's area—Located in the temporal brain region; it is involved with comprehension of auditory and visual information and is necessary for the decoding and encoding of language.

INTRODUCTION

Communication stems from the Latin word *communicare,* "to impart, participate, convey and share information about" (*Webster's New Collegiate Dictionary,* 1974, p. 228). It is the act or reciprocal process of imparting or interchanging thoughts, attitudes, emotions, opinions, or information by speech, writing, or signs. Communication is so greatly rooted in human behaviors and the contexts of society that it is difficult to imagine social or behavioral **transactions** without it. For these reasons communication is fundamental to all nursing and interpersonal relationships. Nurses can use this dynamic and interactive process to motivate, influence, educate, facilitate mutual support, and acquire essential information necessary for survival, growth, and an overall sense of well-being (Howells, 1975; Kleinman, 2004).

Communication also involves performing designated tasks and displaying behaviors such as establishing shared meaning, offering therapeutic instructions, performing client interviews, eliciting relevant data, explaining procedures, educating clients and families, discussing treatment options, describing adverse effects from medications, and providing crisis intervention. Interpersonal skills are by nature relational and process driven, and the consequences of effective communication are **rapport** and trust, acceptance, warmth, **empathy**, support, and stress and anxiety reduction (Duffy et al., 2004).

It is essential for nurses to develop and maintain competent communication and interpersonal skills. As a nurse you must listen empathetically and have a clear understanding of nonverbal and verbal communication skills. Effective communication skills are required to facilitate therapeutic interactions, assess client needs, and implement interventions that promote an optimal level of functioning. This process begins with understanding the instinctive nature of people. Human beings are social and depend on verbal and nonverbal communication to survive and understand internal and external environments. The newborn learns to distinguish and relate to caregivers through facial expression, touching, and feeding. Early forms of communication and interactions with primary caregivers are the origin of trust, security and safety, and lifelong interpersonal relationships and communication patterns (Antai-Otong & Wasserman, 2003). Over time, early interactions with primary caregivers become the foundation of adult relationships, self-esteem, and trust in others. Understanding major principles of effective communication is essential for the nurse because clients and families depend upon these relationships for empathy, reassurance, and quality care to maximize resources and champion positive treatment outcomes.

Increasingly, nurses experience difficulties forming these relationships in today's fast-paced and hurried society. Technological advances in communication processes challenge people to converse through various modes including cellular phones, pagers, various informatics such as video recoding and telehealth, and conference calls, emails, fax technology, chat rooms, and telemedicine. We are frequently inundated with information and communications that must be quickly assimilated, synthesized, analyzed, and correctly interpreted to ensure accurate diagnoses and treatment. Despite efforts to immediately access information, communicate instantaneously, and strive for more efficiency through technological advances, there are growing concerns that information is being shared, but less is communicated. A lack of personal contact or face-to-face interactions contributes to misunderstanding of verbal and written cues. Unquestionably, today's nurse must possess skills that enable her or him to integrate technological advances and computer literacy to ensure effective verbal and nonverbal communication skills. Healthy interactions with clients, families, and other staff are critical in today's fast-paced and information-driven society.

Effective partnerships extend beyond the nurse–client relationship and include collaborative encounters with the interdisciplinary team including physicians, other health care providers, and internal and external customers. Interdisciplinary collaboration has been highlighted as a critical element of quality health care and staff satisfaction. Of particular importance is the nurse–physician relationship. Research findings indicate that effective communication between the nurse and physician enhances problem solving and decision making and improves treatment outcomes (Boyle & Kochinda, 2004; Schmidt & Svarstad, 2002). In contrast, negative or poor communication between the nurse and physician has a deleterious impact on staff morale, staff and client satisfaction, treatment outcomes, and quality of care (Larson, 1999; Rosenstein, 2002; Rosenstein & O'Daniel, 2005). Attempts to maintain effective communication between physicians and nurses must be a priority. Partnerships during a time of dwindling resources, time constraints, and demands for quality care across the continuum just make sense.

In a large survey that examined the prevalence and impact of physicians' disruptive behavior on the job satisfaction and retention of nurses (Rosenstein, 2002; Rosenstein & O'Daniel, 2005), involving 50 Veterans Healthcare Administration hospitals across the country that targeted nurses, physicians, and administrators, researchers discovered that staff had negative perceptions of the impact of physicians' and nurses' disruptive behavior on staff and client satisfaction and treatment outcomes. Data indicated most respondents perceived that disruptive behavior increased workplace stress and worsened nurse–physician communication, information sharing, and workplace relationships. Even more daunting were the respondents' negative perceptions of the effects of these damaging interactions on job satisfaction and staff morale, medication errors, client safety and mortality, and ultimately client satisfaction, clinical outcomes, and quality of care (Rosenstein & O'Daniel). All in all, these data strengthen the argument that healthy nurse–physician relationships are crucial to advancing health care, as well as improving staff morale and treatment outcomes.

The following section focuses on communication theories, modes of communication, and factors that influence communication. It also provides a litany of **therapeutic communication** techniques that enable the nurse to establish rapport, recognize barriers to communication, and develop the mutual trust necessary to gather relevant data, make accurate diagnoses, establish goals, implement client-centered interventions, and facilitate positive treatment outcomes.

COMMUNICATION THEORIES

Effective communicators tailor their message to the knowledge, interest, and abilities of their recipients. They create a climate of openness and trust to facilitate relationships. They are actively engaged and utilize all senses to assess and evaluate verbal and nonverbal cues to ensure accurate understanding of the message. This reciprocal process involves both the nurse and the client as both senders and receivers of messages throughout the interaction. Astute observational and active listening skills enable the nurse to accurately analyze verbal and nonverbal cues and respond appropriately.

Although many people associate communication with verbal messages or words, nonverbal communication has the most powerful influence on interpersonal relationships. For instance, when the client tells the nurse that he is fine and has no complaints, yet his facial expression such as frowning communicates discomfort, an incongruent message is transmitted. Words must be understood within the context of feelings, emotions, attitudes, and body language. **Body language** refers to nonverbal communication or transmission of a message by way of physical gestures or behaviors. It is imperative to clarify verbal and nonverbal communication even when they are congruent to ensure accurate understanding of the client's message. Further discussion of these concepts is forthcoming in this chapter.

Peplau's Interpersonal Relations Theory

Peplau's seminal publication, *Interpersonal Relations in Nursing* (1952), presented a conceptual framework on the therapeutic process between the nurse and the client. Her work has influenced every aspect of nursing. It is considered the cornerstone of interpersonal relationship theories and the basis of all nurse–client communications. Communication occurs within nurse–client relationships and is influenced by complex factors including environment and early interactions with caregivers or parents, and is based on attitudes, beliefs, and practices within the dominant culture.

Peplau's theory (1952) delineated four phases of the nurse–client relationship. These phases are interrelated and each describes the responsibilities and task of the nurse and the client as one of the following:

- *Orientation*—The client's willingness to seek treatment and trust the nurse is an important aspect of this phase. The client communicates his or her needs as the nurse conveys empathy and caring and attempts to understanding the client's experience. Through clarification of the client's problem and situation the nurse listens attentively as he or she reviews events that require attention. Information sharing, questioning, clarification, attentive listening, and exploration of treatment options provide the basis of the nurse–client relationship. First impressions about the nurse and health care system evolve during the orientation phase and transition through subsequent phases.
- *Identification*—Nurse–client interactions provide the basis for trust, acceptance, understanding, and a helping relationship. Through effective communication the nurse identifies client problems and experiences. This process also enables the client to become an active participant in treatment, minimizes feelings of powerlessness and helplessness, and assures that things will improve. Ultimately, through the nurse–client relationship, the client identifies with and trusts the nurse and other staff to assist during times of anxiety and stress.
- *Exploitation*—Through the nurse–client relationship the client gains a sense of independence and navigates the health care system as an active participant in his or her care. The client learns to exploit the nurse–client relationship to identify treatment goals, galvanize health care resources, and attain an optimal level of functioning.
- *Resolution*—As the client's needs are met through nurse–client partnerships and effective communication, the client moves towards full independence and resolution of health care problems or needs.

Overall, Peplau's theory asserts that the goal of communication is to use symbols or concepts that convey meaning and ease the struggle towards a greater understanding between the nurse and client. The nurse–client relationship challenges the nurse to clarify the meaning or expression of the client's problems and distress and maintain continuity during the conversation when the nurse picks up threads of conversation the client offers during nurse–client interactions. This work will be discussed in depth in Chapter 3.

Dyadic Interpersonal Communication Model

Berlo (1960) coined the term *dyadic interpersonal communication* to describe a dynamic interactive process that comprises a source or sender (encoder), whose aim is to be understood by another person or recipient (decoder), who processes, analyzes and decodes, and comprehends the message. The recipient responds to the message based on his or her interpretation of the message. The feedback process in this model enables the sender to validate or modify messages. Communication occurs within a context influenced by the situation, the message's content, attitude, perception, and the emotional and physical state of the sender and recipient. The clearer the message the more likely it will be understood. This is a very useful model that can help both the novice and experienced nurse (encoder) to communicate using the feedback process to validate accuracy and congruence of verbal and nonverbal messages (see Figure 1-1).

Experiential Communication Theories

An example of experiential communication theory is described in the next by Virginia Satir (1967). Satir (1967), a distinguished family therapist, defined communication as a process of giving and getting information. She further noted that individuals must clearly communicate if they expect others to

  Message

Encoder (sender)   Decoder (recipient)

Figure 1-1 Berlo's dyadic interpersonal communication model.

meet their needs. She stressed the importance of getting one's needs met as essential for survival. Communication must be clear, honest, and direct. This process is defined as **transactions** or interactions, which involve verbal and nonverbal messages. Diverse means are employed to communicate, such as using symbols and clues to transmit and receive messages. Although the intention of communication is clarity, it is impossible to achieve absolutely clear communication. Apart from using communication to meet one's needs and survive, it is also a reliable indicator of psychosocial functioning. Satir's communication theory is similar to other theorists whose work is described as effective or *functional*; this type of communication involves the following steps:

1. Clearly state the message. (Sender sends a message.)
2. Receive verbal responses and nonverbal behavior. (Receiver receives and deciphers the message.)
3. Ask for feedback. (Sender validates the message by conversing with receiver.)
4. Be receptive to feedback. (Sender is willing to clarify message if it is misunderstood or unclear.)

According to Satir, both the sender and the recipient of the message are responsible for clarifying the message. Mutual clarification between parties reduces miscommunication and generalizations and enables them to give evidence of their assumptions and validate the meaning of the message.

Communication occurs within the context of people, places, situations, and other social and interpersonal conditions. Clear and effective communication requires *congruency* between physical gestures or behaviors, such as tone of voice or facial expression, and the spoken language. For example, a wife who says "I love you" in a pleasant tone of voice while smiling and embracing her spouse is sending a congruent message. More than likely the recipient accurately interprets this message. In contrast, *incongruent messages* demonstrate inconsistency between what is said and body language. For instance, a husband who states, "I am fine," yet frowns, grimaces, and avoids eye contact. Clearly, he is not fine and the spouse is unsure what he is communicating.

Ineffective or dysfunctional communicators tend to overgeneralize and fail to send complete messages as noted in the following statements:

I am very . . . you know.
They always . . . well, it's clear what they do.

These speakers rely on the receiver to complete the sentence. Incongruent communicators place an immense burden on the receiver and ultimately impede the feedback process. This enables the ineffective communicator to let others take responsibility for clarifying the message. This often results in miscommunication and jeopardizes the quality of interpersonal relationships.

Communication theories provide a guide to assist the student in understanding the basis of how nurse–client interactions and interventions can engender trust, facilitate problem solving, and stimulate holistic interventions. Today's students and nurses are challenged to integrate various communication theories, including Satir's into changing trends that impact communication through diverse venues and demographics.

The following section focuses on factors and trends associated with communication patterns that facilitate a greater understanding of the human experience of illness and health. The contributions of biological issues, psychosocial and cultural influences, life span and developmental factors, technological advances, and societal and health care trends will also be presented.

FACTORS AND TRENDS ASSOCIATED WITH COMMUNICATION

Communication involves complex biological processes, psychosocial influences, and developmental milestones that occur within the context of societal and health care trends and an explosion of technological advances. Combined, these factors influence how one speaks, what one says, and how people relate to each other both verbally and nonverbally.

The nurse is a matrix of biological, psychosocial, and developmental factors that challenge her or him to interact with clients—who also bring a matrix of lifelong psychosocial experiences and emotional and biological needs—within a social climate that expects them to form therapeutic communication. **Therapeutic communication** refers to a healing or curative relationship between the nurse and others. This concept is consistent with Peplau's classic work (1952), which affirms that both the nurse and client bring with them unique experiences, values, beliefs, and expectations regarding interpersonal relationships. During their encounters communication is both verbal and nonverbal and reflects their core assumptions (Peplau, 1952). Therapeutic interactions afford the nurse and client opportunities to clarify communication and facilitate an optimal state of health. Clarity of communication engenders mutual respect and commitment between the nurse and client. Furthermore, nurse–client encounters facilitate data gathering; analysis, synthesis, and validation of clinical findings; accurate diagnosis; and appropriate treatment. More significantly it promotes understanding and recovery.

Mounting evidence shows that effective communication and mutual sharing are the most important determinants of client satisfaction with care, and that they improve the clinician's sense of competence and confidence. Both adults and children value effective communication because it facilitates mutual trust, respect, and candid discussion that guide staff, clients, and families in challenging care choices (Boise & White, 2004; Winn, Cook, & Bonnel, 2004). Effective communication also is linked to improved adherence to treatment and positive clinical outcomes (Harms et al., 2004; Roter et al., 1997) as well as client recall of information, and it may safeguard against malpractice suits (Levinson & Chaumeton, 1999).

On the whole, communication is a complex process, and now more than ever is requisite to successful nurse–client relationships, client satisfaction, and positive clinical outcomes. Understanding the complexity of communication is critical to recognizing diverse influences that promote and impede healthy nurse–client interactions. Communication is often seen as a natural process, but complex biological processes mediated by psychosocial and cultural influences within a changing society and health care system place inordinate pressure and challenges on today's nurse. The following sections provide an overview of a variety of factors that impact communication and nurse–client relationships.

Biological Issues

Neurobiology of Language and Communication

Although communication extends beyond spoken words or speech, language is an integral part of this process. **Speech** is the motor act of communicating through articulation and verbal expression, whereas **language** is the primary venue of communicating ideas and thoughts. It links nations, societies, cultures, communities, individuals, and history and is the foundation of human intelligence. Language involves both production and comprehension. It is governed by cerebral hemispheric dominance, which is associated with handedness, a trait that seems to be genetically determined. Right-handed individuals show an overwhelming bias towards left-hemispheric speech lateralization (Flagg, Cardy, Roberts, & Roberts, 2005). The left hemisphere controls written and spoken language and math calculations and plays a role in comprehension of sentences and processing information, whereas the right hemisphere comprehends only simple language and primarily is involved in spatial construction and patterns. Generally, areas involved in comprehending speech and written words are housed in the left hemisphere. Damage or lesions in these brain regions often leads to speech-language deficits. For instance, a client who suffers a stroke in the left hemisphere is more likely to experience significantly more language and speech deficits or aphasias than one with a lesion in the right hemisphere.

Speech Centers

Neuroimaging studies from the last 20 years and neuroscientists' investigations have demonstrated that vast, complex, and overlapping brain regions underlie the elements of language and speech (Alberca, Montes, Russell, Gil-Néciga, & Mesulam, 2004; Mesulam, 1990). Primary brain regions involved in speech are located in the sylvian fissure or lateral cerebral sulcus of the categorical hemisphere (see Illustration 1.1). One of these regions is the Wernicke area, which is located at the posterior end of the superior temporal gyrus. The superior temporal gyrus is generally larger on the left side and plays a critical role in supporting language in humans (Foundas, Leonard, Gilmore, Fennell, & Heilman, 1996; Pugh et al., 2001). Neuroimaging studies implicate alterations and abnormal lateralization in the superior temporal

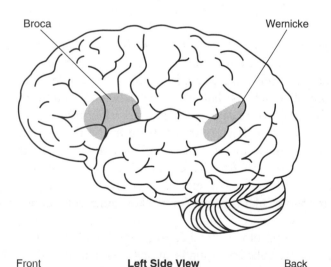

Broca   Wernicke

Front   **Left Side View**   Back

Illustration 1-1 Primary brain regions involved in speech

gyrus as a source of auditory hallucinations in persons with schizophrenia (Levitan, Ward, & Catts, 1999). Wernicke's area is involved with comprehension of auditory and visual information and is necessary for decoding and encoding language. It extends to **Broca's area** in the frontal lobe. Broca's area is involved in the production of speech and articulation and processes information received from Wernicke's area into a complex and synchronized pattern for vocalization; it then projects the pattern through a speech articulation region to the motor cortex, which generates appropriate movements of the lips, tongue, and larynx to initiate speech. In essence, the Wernicke area is responsible for processing incoming speech and the Broca area is responsible for processing outgoing speech.

The auditory cortex also plays a significant role in processing complex sensory information and determines how it is interpreted and integrated. Auditory input is interpreted in the superior temporal gyri and in the inferior parietal lobule and temporal regions previously mentioned. Damage to or deficits in specific brain regions contribute to language deficits and impair one's ability to interpret, understand, or make sense of spoken communication. These conditions interfere with language development and pose significant barriers to the communication process (Alberca et al., 2004; Mesulam, 1990).

Language, Speech, and Learning Disorders

Common language disorders include stuttering, autism, and aphasias. Stuttering is linked to right cerebral dominance and pervasive overactivity of the cerebral cortex and cerebellum. Activation of this region is also associated with the production of laughter—both its duration and its intensity. Clinical features of autism, a neurodevelopmental disorder, include social and communicative deficits that affect the individual's ability to relate to or understand others or to establish reciprocal relationships, as well as repetitive and stereotypical behaviors that emerge in the first 3 years of life and persist throughout adulthood (American Psychiatric Association [APA], 2000).

Aphasias refer to the loss of the ability to comprehend or generate language. Although most aphasias stem from neurological conditions such as cerebral vascular accidents or strokes, other conditions such as brain trauma or injury can also produce these disorders. Symptoms emerge from blockage of a cerebral blood vessel caused by a blood clot or thrombosis. Language deficits are linked to lesion location—whether the lesion is in the dominant or nondominant hemisphere. Aphasias can be classified into two simple types: fluent and nonfluent (Faroqi-Shah & Thompson, 2003; Prather, Zurif, Love, & Brownell, 1997). In *nonfluent* or *expressive* aphasia, the lesion is found in

Broca's area. Clients with this type of aphasia speak slowly and have difficulty generating words and writing. Their verbal comprehension, however, is relatively intact. In comparison, lesions associated with *fluent aphasia* are located in Wernicke's area. Clients with fluent aphasia have normal speech and speak incessantly using neologisms, but the quality of their speech is meaningless; words are often inappropriate and make little sense. These people have disturbance in understanding all language—they fail to comprehend the meaning of spoken or written words (Faroqi-Shah & Thompson; Prather et al.).

The inability to communicate is devastating, and treatment to restore function is valued. Current treatment of aphasia is based on the condition's etiology and includes a holistic approach that integrates cognitive neurorehabilitation, computer-aided techniques, and psychosocial interventions. Major nursing goals for the client with aphasia include supporting physiologic function and working with the interdisciplinary team to ensure holistic interventions that focus on regaining conversational skills and alternative communication. Emotional and psychosocial support and patience are integral elements of treatment. Because of the high incidence of depression due to damage to emotional centers and emotional response in persons with strokes, it is imperative to assess for signs and symptoms of suicide risk.

Dyslexia, a learning disability, is an inability to learn to read. It is found 12 times more often in left-handers, seemingly due to an abnormality in the left hemisphere of the brain that led to a switch in handedness during early development (Ganong, 1999; Shaywitz et al., 2003; Simos, Breier, Fletcher, Bergman, & Papanicolaou, 2000). Findings from a neuroimaging study conducted by Pugh and colleagues (2001) indicated that skilled word identification in reading is associated with the functional integrity of the left hemisphere posterior systems—a dorsal and ventral circuit that comprise temporoparietal and occipitotemporal regions, respectively. Scientists submit that individuals with developmental dyslexia have functional disturbances in these brain regions. In comparison to persons with normal function, persons with dyslexia rely more on both inferior frontal and right hemisphere posterior regions than normally developing readers, probably to compensate for left hemisphere deficits (Pugh et al.; Shaywitz et al.; Simos et al.).

Sensory-Perceptual Influences

Sensations and perceptions are integral aspects of communication and serve as filters for external cues and internal responses. Intact processes facilitate accurate interpretation of verbal and nonverbal communication. Effective listening is often governed by what is in one's head rather than the external world. *Sensory systems* convert external stimuli into neural impulses and then filter irrelevant information to generate an internal image of the external environment, which requires logical reasoning or thinking in higher brain processing regions. These interpretations govern emotions and responses. *Perception* refers to a mental process by which sensory stimuli are brought to consciousness or awareness. The value and degree of comprehension that directs communication determines the ability to synthesize information. Hence, it is imperative for the nurse to have some understanding of the client's functional, mental, and physical status and ability to communicate. Factors such as mental and physical condition, anxiety, stress, and poor listening skills impede accurate interpretation of verbal and nonverbal cues. In addition, conditions that impair attention and concentration play key roles in sensory and perceptual function.

As a rule, the frontal cortex is believed to participate in executive functions, working memory and attention, motivation, cognition, and sensory-perceptual cues. The preservation of attention requires an intact frontal lobe, particularly the right frontal lobe. It mediates and facilitates attention to internal stimuli from key sensory regions, ascribes the relevance of stimuli, and is important for designating appropriate behavioral responses to external and internal stimuli (Buschsbaum, 2004). It also incorporates data from parietal and temporal brain regions with intricate perceptual data from sensory and motor systems to execute cognitive tasks (Buschsbaum).

Damage to or deficits in frontal cortex function impair attention, concentration, and cognitive and communication function. Schizophrenia, depression, attention deficit/hyperactivity disorder (ADHD), and various anxiety disorders such as obsessive-compulsive disorder are examples of psychiatric conditions linked with alterations in frontal lobe function. Alzheimer's disease is also associated with damage or deterioration of the frontal lobe and other brain regions, which causes subsequent sensory-perceptual disturbances (e.g., hallucinations, delusions) as well as problems with speech, attention, concentration, and motor and sensory function including verbal and nonverbal communication. Of these diagnoses, schizophrenia has probably been the most extensively researched. Of particular interest to this discussion are sensory-perceptual symptoms associated with hallucinations in persons with schizophrenia.

Although the precise cause of auditory hallucinations, a cardinal feature of schizophrenia, continues to be debated, mounting evidence from neuroimaging studies indicate that alterations in connectivity between the frontal lobe and temporoparietal speech regions (e.g., superior temporal gyri [Wernicke's area]) may contribute to the pathophysiology of auditory hallucinations (David, 1999; Hubl et al., 2004; Levitan et al., 1999; Slade & Bentall, 2002). Purportedly, during inner speech, persons with schizophrenia experience abnormal coactivation in brain regions associated with language and auditory processing of external stimuli because they are unable to differentiate self-generated thoughts from external stimuli (David; Hubl et al.; Levitan et al.; Slade & Bentall). Alterations in these regions and subsequent sensory-perceptual deficits associated with hallucinations continue to be investigated.

Neurodevelopmental Disorders

Neurodevelopmental disorders, such as autism, produce lifelong disabilities that impact quality of life and ability to communicate and to form meaningful relationships. The exact cause of autism continues to be studied. Although most findings from neuroimaging, behavioral, and neuropsychological studies are tentative, most implicate alterations in genetic vulnerabilities and intricate neuroanatomical regions as contributing to social and behavioral dysfunction distinct to this population (Klin, Jones, Schultz, Volkmar, & Cohen, 2002; Rutter, 2000). Early childhood onset of autism is marked by profound social disability due to poor executive functioning (such as poor attention span and emotional control, reduced impulse control, poor planning, and difficulty moving from one activity to another). Collectively, these behaviors impact the child's capacity to understand or relate to others, express feelings, and establish interpersonal relationships due to social dysfunction and problems with language and communication, learning, and unusual behaviors (APA, 2000).

Biological factors associated with one's ability to speak, express feelings, and form interpersonal relationships are vast. A discussion of these factors is beyond the breadth of this book; however, nurses must be able to distinguish normal versus abnormal factors that promote or impede communication across the life span and implement interventions that facilitate healthy nurse–client interactions and optimal functional status.

Psychosocial Issues

Humans are social beings. There is substantial evidence that adaptation and health status and outcomes are associated with the quality and accessibility of personal relationships. This is particularly relevant to nurses who interact with clients daily and base their interventions and goal setting on the quality of nurse–client relationships. Purportedly, the quality of early infant and child interactions with primary caregivers and ultimately attachment style are reflected in the quality of nurse–client communication patterns and health and adaptation.

Bowlby's (1973) **attachment theory** provides one explanation of normal psychosocial development, adaptation and biological underpinnings, and their potential impact on lifelong communication patterns, people's ability to relate to others, and their willingness to rely on others during stressful periods. His theory suggests that **attachment** is innate and governed by biological processes in the brain that regulate affective or emotionally driven survival behavior.

Simply stated, attachment refers to the interaction and regulation of biological harmony between the infant and primary caregivers. Researchers assert that early secure attachments govern psychobiologic regulatory processes in the infant's developing limbic system—specialized brain areas, mainly in the right hemisphere, adapted to a rapidly developing brain (Schore, 2000). Because the right hemisphere is connected to the limbic and autonomic nervous system, it may play a pivotal role in stress responses and facilitate coping capabilities across the life span (Schore, 2000, 2001). According to attachment theory, cognitive, emotional, and behavioral components underlie secure and insecure attachment styles. The cognitive component is the primary attribute of secure attachments, indicating that the individual has positive concepts of self and trusts others to be responsive during times of need (Bartholomew & Horowitz, 1991; Kidd & Sheffield, 2005). From an emotional perspective, secure attachment style is linked to adaptive coping behaviors, which enable the person to modulate stress and tolerate frustration and other negative emotions. Finally, people with secure attachment styles are at ease with closeness in interpersonal relationships, communicate and express their feelings effectively, and feel comfortable relying on and being comforted by others (Bartholomew & Horowitz; Waters & Cummings, 2000). In contrast, an individual with insecure attachment styles cognitively has negative perceptions of self and others, and has difficulty communicating with and seeking caregiving from others during times of need. Emotionally, these individuals lack the capacity to modulate intense and negative emotions due to maladaptive coping skills, and they are excessively anxious and fearful of closeness. Behaviorally, they tend to be overly clingy or distant and experience fears of abandonment, have difficulty communicating, and find it difficult to form healthy interpersonal relationships (Ainsworth, Blehar, Waters, & Wall, 1978; Bartholomew & Horowitz; Ognibene & Collins 1998; Waters & Cummings).

Memories of early attachment relationships, positive or negative, are communicated through the language of affect (emotional state) and influence the ability to modulate and relate to others across the life span (Amini et al., 1996; Schore, 1997; 2000). Over time, insecure attachment styles contribute to maladaptive coping behaviors and increase vulnerability to illnesses, such as personality, eating, mood, and anxiety disorders (Brennan & Shaver, 1998; Goldberg, 2003; Schore, 1997; West, Rose, Verhoff, Spreng, & Bobey, 1998).

The nurse can help the client communicate more effectively by understanding the reasons underlying cognitive, emotional, and behavioral problems associated with maladaptive coping styles. One approach involves assessing these behaviors and using assertive communication skills to role model emotional competence, foster trust, and form therapeutic interactions. This process begins with **self-awareness** of how one sees oneself and others, and the competence to navigate in the world through positive and healthy relationships. It is imperative to avoid personalizing negative comments or responses because they reflect a repertoire of experiences and perceptions brought in by the client. Negative or rejecting responses reinforce negative perceptions and need to be avoided. The nurse also must be emotionally competent in order to be responsive to the client's emotional and medical needs. **Emotional competence** governs communicative and social functions concerning the individual's ideas, thoughts, motivations, and adeptness at establishing interpersonal relationships (Furr & Funder, 1998; Keltner & Haidt, 2001; Smith & Pope, 1992). Effective modulation or control of negative feelings or emotions is required in order to initiate and maintain close interpersonal relationships and communication. It enables the nurse to listen attentively to the client without bias and remain emotionally present to ensure appropriate responsiveness. A failure to effectively manage one's emotions and adapt to stressful situations threatens the communication process and interpersonal interactions. For example, when an individual is angry and unable to manage the physiological and emotional processes associated with the situation that evoked the anger, he is likely to be controlled by his emotional state and become irrational and out of control, resulting in aggressive and threatening communication. In contrast, the individual who gets angry and controls her emotions—through self-awareness, appropriate control of physiologic and emotional responses, and assertive communication skills—can focus on the issues from an intellectual rather than an emotional perspective and communicate thoughts, feelings, and ideas in a nonthreatening and sociably appropriate manner.

Obviously, communication is vital to healthy human interactions. Understanding various psychosocial factors—including the impact of early relationships with primary caregivers on perceptions of self and others, on the ability to modulate intense and negative emotions, and on the ability to rely on others during times of need—is requisite for effective communication and interpersonal relationships. The nurse must recognize adaptive and maladaptive behaviors within a social context and use nurse–client relationships to enrich and role model healthy interactions. Nurses, like their clients, must recognize the role of their early childhood relationships as well as their attachment styles and their potential impact on nurse–client relationships. Personal awareness enables the nurse to respect and recognize the potential and actual impact of psychosocial issues, coping and attachment styles, emotional responsiveness, and communication with clients across the life span.

The Role of Culture in Communication

The 2000 U.S. Census confirmed that this country is more diverse than ever before (U.S. Census Bureau, 2000). More than ever, the client's perception of health and expectations for care, treatment options, and health practices parallel his or her socioeconomic status, culture, ethnicity, gender, and religious beliefs.

Communication and language are initial challenges when client interactions involve diversity (Kavanagh & Kennedy, 1992). Converging evidence also indicates that the sociocultural differences between clinicians and clients influence communication, diagnosis, and clinical decision making (Berger, 1998; Einbinder & Schulman, 2000; Flores, 2000; Office of Minority Health, 2001; Street, 2002). It is important to note, however, that cultures are not homogeneous. Assorted factors, such as degree of acculturation, age, education, socioeconomic status, family structure, religion, spirituality, gender, and country of origin modify the impact of one's culture and ethnicity and influence expression of distress, health beliefs and practices, and perception of health and illness (Kagawa-Singer & Kassim-Lakha, 2003).

Appreciation of the impact of culture on the client and treatment outcomes is "essential for well-being, growth, survival . . ." (Leininger, 2002, p. 192). Nurses must bridge the gap between themselves and their clients through cultural competence. Every culture characterizes health for its members; delineates acceptable health practices, communication patterns, and language and expression; and defines how to adapt to distress (Leininger, 2002). It also enables individuals to restore and maintain a sense of well-being. The communication process becomes more significant during distressful situations because they often require health education, appreciation of diversity, partnerships with the client and family, and accurate explanations of procedures and their psychological and physical ramifications. The nurse must also take into account educational level, language, and literacy when communicating with clients and families from diverse cultural and ethnic backgrounds (Munet-Vilaró, 2004).

Failure to consider sociocultural factors when communicating with *all* clients may result in stereotyping, mistrust, biased and inaccurate diagnoses, and inappropriate treatment of clients based on culture, ethnicity, language, race, or social status (Antai-Otong, 2002; van Ryn & Burke, 2000). Numerous studies show that clients from racial and ethnic minority groups are less likely to have a positive perception of providers or to trust providers than are other groups (Cooper-Patrick et al., 1999; Murray-Garcia, Selby, Schmittdiehl, Grumbach, & Quesenberry, 2000; Taira et al., 1997). A lack of trust erodes the nurse–client relationship. Trust is nurtured through acceptance, empathy, sensitivity, and a willingness to glean a greater understanding of client symptoms, communication patterns, health practices, and belief systems. The nurse can further strengthen trust and rapport by embracing family strengths and uniqueness and appreciating their level of distress, as reflected by client-centered care (Antai-Otong; Cioffi, 2003).

Culturally sensitive communication is every client's right. It requires empathy, self-awareness, respect, concern, and humility. These are basic aspects of nursing. Regardless of the client's culture, race, socioeconomic status, or ethnicity, *all* require individualized health care free of bias and stereotyping and an approach that encourages expression of feelings, thoughts, and attitudes and participation in client-centered care.

As previously mentioned, positive health outcomes and client satisfaction are closely linked with responsiveness to the client's wishes, preferences, and needs (Brown, Boles, Mullooly, & Levinson, 1999). Owing to the potential deleterious impact of biased and inappropriate care on treatment outcomes, efforts to use culturally sensitive communication skills are a priority. Although there is tentative data that indicate a failure to provide culturally sensitive communication and health care is likely to result in negative outcomes and distrust, it is vital for researchers to move beyond awareness to identifying and implementing communication strategies that help nurses respond more effectively to culturally diverse populations. An in-depth discussion of nurse–client interactions will be discussed in Chapter 4, Cultural Aspects of Communication Partnerships.

Developmental/Life Span Issues

Infancy and Childhood

Communication throughout the life span is essential for health and survival. It is well-documented that infants given minimal physical care in institutions or homes fail to thrive and their development and well-being are compromised. In comparison, holding, stroking, smiling, feeding, soothing, and caring for babies promote normal growth and development and a sense of well-being. Neuroimaging studies strengthen this premise and indicate early environmental sensory input shapes the brain's neural structures, which serve as the underpinnings of the mind and personality. Purportedly, within hours after birth the infant is visually sensitive to the caretaker's face; within days he or she recognizes the mother's voice and within weeks he or she favors the mother's face. Parents and caregivers who create sensory environments using various means of communication may be able to shape vast high-level cognitive and motor structures associated with thinking, planning, coping, and modulating anxiety and stress. A failure to shape these neural structures through positive early sensory communication may result in lifelong difficulty modulating anxiety and stress (Sinha, Lacadie, Skudlarski, & Wexler, 2004).

Because of the potential positive and negative impacts of early interactions between the infant and primary caregivers, it is useful to use John Bowlby's attachment theory, discussed earlier in the chapter, to explain the infant's developmental perspective. Attachment refers to a lasting affectional tie or emotional bond initially between the infant and primary caregivers, and involves seeking closeness to one or more caregivers to feel safe and secure, and provide a means of understanding the world (Ainsworth, Blehar, Waters, & Wall, 1978; Bowlby, 1969, 1973, 1980). Secure attachment fosters independence and mastery of the environment and exploration of the child's surroundings from a stable foundation provided by primary caregivers.

Secure attachments styles during infancy generally result in healthy communication and interpersonal skills in adulthood. The attachment theory links secure attachment styles in adults to specific positive interactions during infancy with primary caregivers (Collins & Feeney, 2000; Ognibene & Collins, 1998). Early secure attachments also contribute to the neurophysiology of the developing brain, specifically the right hemisphere, during its peak growth period (Amini et al., 1996; Schore, 2001). Secure attachment styles and communication are demonstrated in children who are sensitive and receptive to caregiving (Ainsworth et al., 1978). They are playful, happy, and receptive to affection expressed by primary caregivers. In comparison, failure to form close and secure attachments during early infancy interferes with establishing close, secure, and safe interpersonal relationships and results in *insecure attachments styles* in adulthood (Bowlby, 1973). Infants and children exposed to inconsistent, harsh, neglectful primary caregivers often experience fears of abandonment and appear frightened, excessively clingy, and anxious and have difficulty communicating their needs.

The enormous task of language development and communication varies throughout the life span, but never more than during early childhood. Language plays a vital role in human learning, communication, and memory. It also is the core of all interpersonal relationships and is reinforced through early interactions with and imitation of parents and primary caregivers. Through early interactions children learn to communicate feelings, attitudes, and ideas; allay fears; understand themselves and others; and form common bonds between themselves and others.

Early speech and communication during infancy occurs with various sensory and perceptual stimuli. The voice and touch of caregivers or parents are crucial for emotional and central nervous system development. Feeding provides nourishment and fulfills oral needs during early infancy and childhood and builds trust, closeness, and a sense of well-being—key factors that promote mental and physical health as well as communication between the child and parents or caregivers. Early interactions foster trust and love and underlie communication across the life span. During the early developmental stages infants and adults also communicate with eye tracking that evokes various nonverbal and verbal communication forms such as smiles, cooing, facial expressions, suckling, crying, grabbing, and kicking. Language production during the first year of life involves coos in response to voice babbling and imitation of sounds (Schwartz, 1990). Towards the end of the first year, the child uses words such as mama/dada meaningfully, and in time true speech emerges. By age 2, 20% of speech is understandable by strangers (Schwartz). Most children across various cultures master all levels of language by age 4 to 5 years.

Adults process speech incrementally, promptly distinguishing spoken words based on initial phonetic information sufficient to discerning them from alternatives. Some researchers submit that during the second year of life infants are capable of incremental speech processing even prior to developing a large vocabulary (Fernald, Swingley, & Pinto, 2001). Lexical or vocabulary growth is also associated with increased speed and efficiency in comprehending oral speech.

Language and communication problems that occur during childhood require knowledge of complex underlying neurobiologic, social, cultural, and family issues. These factors provide a frame of reference of trust, communication and interpersonal skills, self-esteem, and learning. Major challenges emerge when children present in various clinical settings with their parents or caregivers and are unable to express their feelings, communicate effectively, form interactions with family members and peers, maintain attention, manage impulses, and appropriately modulate emotions.

Language difficulties or disorders during this developmental stage may go unrecognized because parents often complete sentences and interpret for the child. Sometimes asking closed-ended sentences elicit yes or no answers. Children presenting with language and speech disorders often misunderstand questions or may expect the nurse to fill in gaps as parents have to make sense of their responses or communication. Treatment issues involving children with language and communication disorders or problems require accurate comprehensive psychiatric, academic, and developmental evaluation to rule out psychiatric conditions, including family history of psychiatric and medical conditions, health practices, and family dynamics.

Clearly, early speech and language delay should cause concern for parents and nurses because it may be a manifestation of comorbid conditions, such as hearing loss, developmental and behavioral disorders, and psychosocial deprivation (Noterdaeme, Mildenberger, Minow, & Amorosa, 2002; Weisbrot & Carlson, 2005). Early identification of speech and language problems is crucial, and with appropriate interventions may allay the emotional, social, behavioral, and cognitive deficits of these disabilities and increase quality of life and self-esteem (Weisbrot & Carlson).

Adolescence

Like childhood, adolescence is an overtaxing period of great transition and reorganization. Adolescents struggle to resolve tremendous biologic changes, psychosocial pressures, and developmental milestones. Peer pressure, the need to belong, and a struggle for self-identity separate the adolescent from parents or caregivers; influence self-image, self-esteem, and sexual identity; and contribute to emotional turbulence. Communication during this period often reflects the language of peers, society, and family. Feelings and thoughts may be communicated through various venues such as music, clothes or fashion, computer games, emails, chat rooms, cellular phones, text messages, snail mail, and family gatherings.

Adolescents are often challenging because of trust issues with adults and the need to separate from family of origin, reflective of interpersonal relationships with parents. Baffled at being between childhood and adulthood, adolescents are usually overly sensitive to criticism and worry that others will disapprove of them, particularly if they have a problem. Poor impulse control, immature thinking processes, and "here and now" thinking make it arduous for the youth to see beyond today. Successful communication with the adolescent requires patience, understanding of developmental milestones including infancy and childhood issues, and a knowledge of the history of the client's and family's medical and psychiatric conditions and family dynamics (see Table 1-1).

Adulthood

Adulthood has been discussed throughout this chapter, and so will not be discussed again in this section.

Older Adulthood

The aging process vastly impacts communication. Normal age-related changes and developmental issues impact the older adult's ability to form nurse–client relationships and cope with aging. Age-related changes in sensory and perceptual processes such as hearing and seeing impact communication because they also influence interpretation of external cues and internal responses. An older adult with visual deficits is likely to misinterpret environmental stimuli and experience more illusions and fears. Illusions are misinterpretations of environmental stimuli—such as when an older person with visual deficits enters a dimly lit room and thinks that a shadow is a person or ghost. In reality the individual is not "seeing things," but misinterpreting environmental stimuli. Adequate lighting and glasses are likely to reveal a shadow versus a ghost or person. When older adults communicate these events and express anxiety and

Table 1-1 Essential Nurse Characteristics

• Establish trust	• Provide explanations for questions
• Be honest and nonjudgmental	• Praise for healthy behaviors and adaptive
• Convey empathy and concern	• Assess level of dangerousness to self and
• Use congruent verbal and nonverbal cues	others
• Discuss confidentiality	• Talk to parents or caregivers
• Use nonthreatening questions	

fears, it is imperative for the nurse to reassure and educate about age-related changes and their impact on sensory-perceptual processes. They often require devices that enhance declining sensory function, including prescription eyeglasses and hearing aids. In addition to sensory-perceptual changes, some older adults may process information more slowly and respond less spontaneously than younger age groups, and also feel threatened by these changes. Communication with older adults requires patience and sensory-enhancing tools or strategies, such as speaking loud, without yelling; using short explanations for those with short-term memory problems; pausing for responses; and using touch and respectful mannerisms appropriately (see Table 1-2).

Lifelong positive experiences, achievements, coping styles, and self-esteem influence developmental issues in older adults and play pivotal roles in their ability to communicate with others during stressful and nonstressful periods. Normal developmental issues impacting communication in the older adult are mediated by age-related changes, cultural influences, values, health practices, and belief systems. Culture and ethnicity impact the older adult's communication skills and language and parallel generational issues such as the need for independence, a sense of "weakness" or dependence, and a need for integrity, dignity, meaningfulness of life, and self-worth (Erikson, 1963). A sense of despair and disgust (Erikson) stems from unsuccessful coping skills related to early childhood issues and ineffective coping styles across the life span, which are detrimental to the client's ability to express feelings, seek help, and communicate with the nurse and other staff.

Intergenerational communication involving older adults is likely to be influenced by the nurse's assumptions about aging, culture and ethnicity, and economic, social, and political systems. It is important to address clients respectfully and avoid using patronizing words such as "sweetie" or "honey" when working with older adults. Cultural influences also determine which personal experiences are communicated and shared with the nurse, and how they are shared. Story-telling is an example of a common form of communication among various cultures, particularly among elder members of the family. Story-telling enables older adults to link the present with the past and

Table 1-2 Major Barriers to Effective Communication with Older Adults

• Ageism or stereotyping	• Sense of futility
• Lack of appreciation for lifelong experiences and meaningfulness in life	• Over identification
• Hurried unconcerned approach	• An overall lack of respect for older adults

ascribe significance to the family legacy. It provides important information about family history, roles, customs, coping styles, and health practices. Taking the time to listen and approaching the client in an unhurried manner are important interventions for the client who needs extra time to respond to queries and are crucial to the nurse–client interaction in this age group. Culture and ethnicity play key roles in how older adults are viewed by family members and communities. It is imperative to respect each older adult as an individual and create relationships that convey respect, appreciation of age-related physical changes, and dignity and preserve integrity.

Communication with older adults is further complicated by various non-age-related medical conditions that cause severe cognitive deficits, such as Alzheimer's disease (AD). Because of deterioration of various brain regions and alteration in biochemistry, the client is unable to process or integrate information and suffers from complex language difficulties including aphasia and/or inability to generate speech.

Data from several studies indicate that despite severe cognitive deficits associated with AD, the client still has a sense of self-awareness (Mayhew, Acton, Yauk, & Hopkins, 2001; Moore & Hollett, 2003; Tappen, Williams, Fishman, & Touhy, 1999). Because it is impossible to ascertain the degree of mental capacity and cognitive deficits of persons with AD it is imperative to treat the client as though he or she understands. Normally, this requires tailoring communication to meet the needs of the client based on mental status and physical findings. Basic communication guidelines include introducing yourself, explaining procedures, making eye contact, calling the person by name, being comfortable with long pauses, orienting the client, and using a warm and pleasant tone of voice. In general, these interventions preserve dignity and convey respect, reverence, compassion, and caring. Nurses must educate families and caregivers about the importance of talking, listening, and respecting the client despite communication and language difficulties. Additional suggestions for improving communication between the caregiver and the client with severe dementia include simplifying vocabulary, using concrete content, speaking slowly, keeping a congenial and pleasant voice tone, and using closed-ended questions (Frank, 1994; Shulman & Mandel, 1993; Tappen, Williams-Burgess, Edelstein, Touhy, & Fishman, 1997).

Communication with persons with severe dementia such as AD is often regarded as incoherent and meaningless. This is particularly devastating to clients and their families. Studies illustrate that the family or caregiver's inability to communicate with clients with cognitive deficits generates feelings of helplessness and purposelessness and suggest that improved communication could diminish or prevent the meaninglessness associated with caring for older adults with severe dementia (Mayhew, Acton, Yauk, & Hopkins, 2001; Sheldon, 1994; Shulman & Mandel, 1993). Negative assumptions about the inability of persons with AD to communicate also threaten their integrity and sense of self and well-being.

Societal and Health Care Trends

Societal trends involving reduced staff, dwindling health care resources, and pressures to provide quality care with fewer dollars challenge nurses to create innovative strategies to communicate effectively with clients. Nurses are the chief providers of health care and are in pivotal positions to advance these strategies and promote healthy interactions. Healthy nurse–client relationships are essential to successful utilization of resources, client satisfaction, and quality care. Through effective interdisciplinary teamwork the nurse orchestrates health care, advocates for quality health care and client rights, and allocates resources and implements interventions that facilitate positive treatment outcomes.

Technological and Information Systems

In 2001, the Institute of Medicine (IOM) felt the growing complexity of science and technology were becoming an essential aspect of quality and safe health care (IOM, 2001). The past few years have seen a plethora of information technologies introduced into hospitals, communities, and homes. Numerous outcome studies show that some technologies improve communication among providers (Bernstein, Farinelli, & Merkatz, 2005), disease management, and self-care management via home monitoring devices and telephone contact (Papazissis, 2004). One such telecommunication technology is telemedicine, which is the use of telecommunication technology to diagnose, monitor, and provide therapeutic intervention when distance separates the client and care provider. This telecommunication approach captures and quickly transmits textual, audio, and video data in rural areas, homes, and other sites where nurses and other staff are not readily accessible (Agency for Healthcare Research and Quality [AHRQ], 2001). Because rapid advances in technology may have the potential to deteriorate the nurse–client relationship, the nurse must be proactive and implement interventions that maintain the quality of these relationships.

Technological advances and the Internet continue to afford opportunities for communication. Nowadays, clients are more knowledgeable about their health care needs, preferences, and alternative therapies and demand nurse–client interactions that are safe, client-centered, culturally and developmentally sensitive, and cost-effective. As a result of technology and Internet access, clients can go online and access various tests, and provide input that allows clinicians to monitor and trend vital signs, weight, wounds, oxygen saturation, and glucose levels and important various medical aspects of chronic disease management. Through diverse interactive communication modalities they can let the nurse know how they are doing, receive psychoeducation, and participate in self-help groups. Overall, researchers submit that the Internet offers numerous opportunities to enhance communication and access to information for clinicians, clients, and other stakeholders (National Research Council, 2000). Meanwhile, privacy and confidentiality, ethical issues, and legal concerns involving access to data via the Internet continue to be debated.

Even as societal and health care trends and technological advances challenge today's nurses, effective communication remains the basis of nursing care. It facilitates trust and understanding and increases sensitivity to the client's experiences and responses across the life span. Linking these changes to diverse modes of communication enhances the quality of nurse–client interactions and facilitates holistic and individualized health care.

MODES OF COMMUNICATION

When we think of communicating, we often envision ourselves talking. Of course, real communication means talking, listening, thinking, interacting, planning, and responding, simultaneously. It means understanding from another person's perspective and interpreting and responding based on personal experiences. The nurse–client interaction requires all the nurse's senses, attention, interest, and competence to analyze behavioral and emotional responses within the context of a given interaction. Modes of communication are influenced by the nurse's adeptness at establishing rapport, trust, and empathy and using active listening as a means of facilitating healthy nurse–client relationships.

The following factors influence effective communication:

- Rapport
- Trust
- Empathy

- The manner in which the message is delivered
- Anxiety and stress
- Language (spoken or verbal communication)
- Body language (nonverbal communications)
- Space

Rapport

Rapport is a harmonious, empathetic, and mutually respectful relationship between the nurse and client. Generally, the nurse is the helping part of the nurse–client relationship. Rapport requires a warm, accepting, confidential, and secure environment that engenders trust, encourages expression of feelings, improves decision-making skills, requires active listening, and promotes healthy and adaptive lifestyle changes. Rapport is necessary for the client to feel comfortable and less anxious and fearful, so he or she can freely express feelings.

The following statement is an example of what a nurse may say to initiate rapport:

> Good morning Mr. Jones, my name is Lisa and I am your nurse today. I understand that this is your first visit. How can I help you today?

The nurse's introduction and subsequent question convey a genuine interest in the client's well-being. Addressing the client by name conveys respect, thoughtfulness, and empathy. This unhurried and caring approach mitigates the client's fears and normal anxiety associated with a first visit, opens lines of communication, and facilitates expression of feelings.

The following is an example of a dialogue that can foster rapport:

Nurse: Good afternoon, Mrs. Chamberlain, my name is Ken; I understand you're upset about the delay in getting your prescription. I'm sorry for the delay and I am waiting for a call from pharmacy. How can I help you right now?

Client: This is the second time this has happened and I am tired of waiting several hours each time I come to the clinic.

Nurse: I understand. I can see you're pretty upset. As soon as I hear from the pharmacist I can tell you how long you have to wait. We will get your prescription as soon as possible.

Client: I feel better knowing that someone is at least trying to help me. I really appreciate your time. I'll just wait until you return. Thank you very much.

The nurse established rapport with this angry client by approaching her in an unhurried manner, immediately expressed understanding, communicated empathy, and avoided defensiveness. The use of active listening skills is a vital component of rapport. Active listening with empathy and impartiality helped the client stay calm and develop a positive relationship with the nurse and staff. A failure to communicate or establish rapport, especially in challenging situations, may escalate the situation and reduce both confidence in the nurse and staff and client satisfaction.

Trust

Trust is germane to therapeutic and authentic nurse–client relationships. Frequently nursing research links trust to human development and healthy ego formation, referring to the contributions of Erikson (1963). Carl Rogers (1977) coupled trust with power, and an environment of openness. Trust indicates that one person can rely or depend on another to follow through on a promise or obligation. Trust stems from consistent, reliable, and positive experiences with early childhood primary caregivers and subsequent adult relationships. Trust is very difficult to engender when the client has a history of poor interpersonal relationships. Normally, nurses experience a high degree of trust in their interactions with clients they serve. This unique position can be used to strengthen trust, foster hope, empower clients to make adaptive changes, and influence quality of life throughout the life span.

As just mentioned, the client's capacity to trust is governed by early interactions with parents and caregivers. However, trust evolves through nurse–client relationships that convey acceptance, empathy, caring, and understanding. As the nurse approaches the client, she or he must use congruent body language and verbal communication, such as good eye contact, extension of hand to greet the client, calmness, and a normal voice tone. For example, when you take a client's vital signs, this process involves greeting the client with good eye contact, calling the client by name, displaying competence to perform the task, and asking him or her which arm he or she prefers for blood pressure. This brief interaction demonstrates respect, acceptance, and caring. Through eye contact and greeting the client by name, the nurse conveys "I accept and respect you as an individual and I am here to help you." By asking which arm he or she prefers for blood pressure reading, the nurse allows the client to participate in decision making. Each nurse–client encounter must be used to convey competence, acceptance, caring, and understanding—the basis of trust. Major nursing attributes that engender trust include:

- Competence
- Reliability
- Confidence
- Hope
- Motivation
- Predictability
- Empathy

- Trustworthiness
- Genuineness and authenticity
- Consistency
- Responsibility
- Conscientiousness
- Kindness
- Fairness

Overall, trust facilitates healthy and effective communication through rapport and nurse–client interactions. It conveys competence and confidence and creates a caring, compassionate, and therapeutic environment of mutual respect, empathy, cooperation, and sincerity.

Empathy

Empathy refers to sharing the feelings, thoughts, and ideas of another. It allows for emotional connectedness and understanding without the experience becoming the nurse's. It is the cornerstone of nursing and determines how the nurse accepts, values, and seeks to understand the client's experiences. It allows the nurse to glean the client's experiences and world through the client's lens. Empathy engenders understanding of the client's feelings and communicates this understanding to the client. By embracing the client's viewpoint the nurse is more likely to see situations or problems as the client does. It is being able to "walk a mile in someone's shoes" without their experience becoming your own. Empathy differs from **sympathy**, in that the latter involves taking on another's experiences and making them yours. For example, after the loss of his wife of 45 years, Mr. Jones feels sad and lost. He talks to you and expresses sadness and grief. *Empathy* enables you to respond to his grief by saying "I understand this is a very difficult time for you." In comparison, *sympathy* is displayed by saying "I feel sad too and want to cry with you." In the latter case the nurse has problems distinguishing her grief from the client's, and hence becomes less effective and objective in facilitating the grief process. Characteristics of sympathy include over-identification with the client's situation, feelings, and thoughts; difficulty removing oneself from the client's experience; and rescuing the client instead of encouraging the client to resolve grief or problems. Although both concepts convey compassion, sympathy is nontherapeutic and compromises the client's grief process and the nurse–client relationship.

The therapeutic nature of empathy lies in "being with the client" but not "becoming the client." This is often difficult for the novice nurse, due to a lack of self-awareness and problems distinguishing personal reactions from the client's. Fortunately, with time, personal development, and self-awareness or insight, the novice nurse will master this essential nursing skill.

The Manner in Which the Message Is Delivered

Communication is a complex process mediated by emotions, attentiveness, understanding, and empathy. It involves both verbal and nonverbal processes that must be congruent; otherwise, the recipient may misinterpret the message and respond accordingly. Self-awareness of our communication styles and patterns and how others perceive us is crucial to understanding ourselves. For instance, if the client asks, "Why are you so angry today?" and your response is "I am not angry" it is essential for you to assess why the client perceived you as being angry. You may not be angry, but something about your tone of voice, use of words, or nonverbal communication led the client to believe you were angry. This is particularly significant if more than one person asks the same question, which generally means that the queries are justifiable. During these occasions it is important to ask reasons for these perceptions, to explore reasons why you may or may not be angry, or just to look in the mirror and assess for cues that may indicate anger. Acknowledging anger is not a sign of weakness because it indicates that strong emotions were outside your radar screen (**self-awareness**). Situations like this also expand self-awareness, decrease defensiveness, and enable you to understand your own emotions and nonverbal cues and determine ways to acknowledge and manage them effectively. Self-awareness refers to personal recognition of one's attitudes, ideas, biases, values, and beliefs that affect relationships with others.

Anxiety and Stress

Emotions play a pivotal role in how a message is delivered. Anxiety and stress can be overwhelming in some cases and interfere with the ability to process information accurately, resulting in the receiver tuning out the message. Anxiety and other emotions are often expressed by gestures, attitude, eye contact, tone of voice, touch, emotional state, facial expressions, and posture. The higher the emotional state the less accurately one hears or communicates messages. An inability to understand messages due to anxiety and stress impedes effective communication, compromises decision making, and prevents appropriate behavioral and verbal responses. For instance, if a nurse is upset or fearful or experiences overwhelming stressors, although she may use appropriate spoken words, the message is likely to be overshadowed or diluted by her emotional state and an incorrect message will be conveyed. Another example is when a client walks into a primary care clinic or is admitted to a surgical unit and feels frightened about his condition; he may appear angry and respond abruptly. If the nurse fails to recognize underlying fears or anxiety, she or he may respond similarly, by speaking loudly or abruptly, hence losing an opportunity to establish rapport, remain calm, reassure the client, and assess the client's needs. During stressful encounters it is imperative for the nurse to:

- Pay close attention to the message.
- Focus on themes and content rather than on how the message is delivered.
- Remain open-minded and objective.
- Clarify and restate what he or she hears before responding.

Equally important, the nurse needs to examine personal feelings toward specific clients and recognize their potential impact on verbal and nonverbal communication with them. Obviously, certain situations and client behaviors make it arduous to create these environments because they are threatening and require patience, self-control, perseverance, knowledge, and maintenance of personal safety.

The following scenario demonstrates the impact of emotions on the nurse–client relationship when the client uses threatening or aggressive behaviors that engender fear in the nurse. Clearly the nurse is frightened, but it is essential for her to respond assertively and set limits to prevent escalation and maintain personal safety.

Client (yelling): No one cares how long it's taken me to drive to this hospital because everyone is busy!

Nurse: Mr. Irvin, I understand you are upset, but it is difficult for me to help when you are yelling and threatening. I will do whatever I can to assist you, but it is important for you to lower your voice.

Client: I'm sorry, but this is the third time I've had to come to the emergency room this month and I don't know what's wrong with me.

> **Nurse:** Mr. Jones, I understand and believe you have reasons to be upset. What brought you in today or what can I do to assist you now?

The client now settles down and becomes more conciliatory. Obviously he was unable to convey his feelings appropriately because of underlying fears and high anxiety levels. The nurse's response and tone of voice were instrumental in mitigating the client's fears and anxiety. Her reassuring mannerisms, assertive communication, and firm and clear limit setting enabled her to ensure personal safety and form a trusting nurse–client interaction. Personal safety must be a priority in situations involving threatening or potentially dangerous situations.

Verbal and Nonverbal Behaviors

Spoken or oral communication has been extensively discussed in this chapter. It is an important part of communication, but has less impact on the meaning of what is said than nonverbal behaviors or cues. For the purposes of this discussion, nonverbal behavior or communication will be referred to as **body language**. The more congruency between verbal and nonverbal communication, the more accurately the message will be interpreted or understood.

Often body language or nonverbal behaviors convey what the person has difficulty saying or articulating. Common body language gestures include eye contact, facial expressions such as frowning or grimacing, tone of voice, hand waving or pointing, head movements, physical appearance and hygiene, general posture and gait, laughter, smiling, and head nodding. The body is a mediator of messages and often uses muscle tone and posture as modes of nonverbal communication (Sloan, Bradley, Dimoulas, & Lang, 2002). For example, the extent one allows oneself to relax during conversations communicates a message. Tense muscles and posture indicate dislike, anxiety, or stress; in contrast, a person who leans toward the respondent and has relaxed facial muscles and a firm handshake indicates he or she is at ease.

Sometimes nonverbal communication occurs simultaneously with verbal communication, and at times the speaker is unaware of these nonverbal signals. Common consequences of incongruent verbal and nonverbal behaviors are miscommunication or misinterpretation of cues. Just because someone smiles does not necessarily mean she or he is happy. In fact, smiling often masks negative or overwhelming emotions, such as fear and anxiety. It is imperative to validate or clarify one's interpretation of these gestures to ensure accuracy of their meaning and avoid responding inappropriately; for example, it is imperative to refrain from smiling inappropriately during interactions because when the client shares important information and the nurse smiles this could be mistaken as "being funny" and belittling or devaluing. Again, self-awareness and how one responds with nonverbal cues is just as important as validating the client's behaviors.

Space

We all know what it feels like when someone invades our **personal space** or "comfort zone." If we feel anxious and uncomfortable when this occurs, just imagine how our clients feel, particularly those who are already anxious and feel threatened. The need for personal distance and space must be recognized and afforded by the nurse. Hall (1966) coined the concept of personal space in interpersonal interactions in his book *The Hidden Dimension*. He asserted that the distance and relevance of space between people is governed by cultural influences. He delineated four principal space distance zones maintained by healthy middle-class Americans, acknowledging that the distance zones are not applicable to all cultures or ethnic populations. He further posited that the specific distance selected is governed by the nature of transactions and relationships between parties—their feelings and actions.

The four distance zones are:

1. *Intimate distance*—Close range and the presence of another person is unmistakable. This is illustrated in love-making, hugging a child, friend, or relative, or holding an infant.
2. *Personal distance*—Ranges from $1\frac{1}{2}$ to 4 feet. Normally this is arm's length.
3. *Social distance*—Ranges from 4 to 12 feet. At this distance parties have minimum if any physical contact and are at a more formal business distance, which is maintained at a staff meeting, supermarket cashier, conference table, or receptionist area.
4. *Public distance*—Ranges from 12 to 25 feet or more, with minimal eye contact. This takes place when walking through a shopping mall or passing someone in the hallway. There is mutual respect to maintain distance and remain strangers. (Hall 1966, 1989)

Caring for clients often forces the nurse to invade the client's personal space (e.g., taking vital signs, changing dressings, providing treatment). It is important to note that the closer the proximity between the nurse and client, the higher the risk of violence or difficulty escaping if necessary. It is imperative for the nurse to be cognizant of his or her own comfort distance zones and appreciate and respect those of clients and staff. Although cultural influences govern people's comfort zones, medical and psychiatric conditions may also influence how one defines one's personal space. Persons with schizophrenia and other severe psychiatric conditions often feel anxious and uncomfortable when the nurse invades their personal space. Increased anxiety also increases the risk of violence—a gesture to protect oneself from harm. In comparison, persons with bipolar disorder during a manic phase may be intrusive and invade the nurse's personal space, requiring the nurse to step back and set limits. Maintain leg's length distance and avoid touching or making sudden movements when caring for clients who are cognitively impaired, suspicious, paranoid, or psychotic. Invading their personal space increases the risk of physical harm and danger. Maintaining a safe distance ensures quick and safe escape. The personal meaning of space is individual, but the nurse must be aware of her comfort distance zone and value and respect those of clients and colleagues.

CRITICAL THINKING QUESTION

Question: What do you do when a client invades your personal space by either hugging or embracing you?

Answer: Your response will vary and depend upon the nature of your relationship with the client or staff. For example, if you have worked with a client and family for several months or years and established a therapeutic relationship, and everyone understands and respects personal boundaries, during a death or very stressful event hugging may be appropriate. There must be mutual acceptance of the behaviors, however. In another situation where the nurse does not know the client or the client is threatening or overly seductive, it is imperative to maintain a safe distance and set firm verbal limits to ensure easy access to an exit to maintain personal safety.

In conclusion, modes of communication are vast. Each nurse must understand him- or herself in order to relate to and understand the client's experience and behavior. A further discussion of the nurse–client relationship will be included in Chapter 3.

LEGAL AND ETHICAL CONSIDERATIONS

Legal and ethical considerations are an integral part of nursing. All information or data gathered during client encounters and interventions with clients is confidential. This includes ensuring confidentiality and privacy, maintaining secure medical records, documenting accurate information in the client's record that can be supported by observations and interpretation, assuring third-party safety, and maintaining professional nurse–client boundaries.

Confidentiality

Nurses are responsible for maintaining confidentiality of information shared by clients and families with the nurse and treatment planning team (Barloon, 2003). The American Nurses Association (ANA) *Code of Ethics for Nurses* (ANA, 2000) states nurse practice acts, and institutions have statements about confidentiality. The registered nurse is encouraged to practice under the auspices of the ANA *Code of Ethics* to guide practice and to:

- Deliver nursing care that preserves and protects client autonomy, dignity, rights, and respect.
- Ensure client confidentiality.
- Demonstrate self-care.
- Serve as client advocate and contribute to resolving ethical issues.
- Maintain a professional client–nurse relationship with appropriate boundaries.

Such statements represent a consensus of general standards of professional conduct. Clients trust the nurse to listen attentively; document in the medical record, and safeguard shared information. It is imperative to keep records out of public reach, including loose papers that need to be shredded rather than tossed in the wastebasket; to avoid discussing a client on the elevator, in a waiting room, or at a work station; and to not leave a computer unlocked or unattended.

Information shared must be used for treatment purposes only unless the client provides written permission to do otherwise. Only when the client provides written permission that specifies what information and how it will be used and to whom it will be shared, usually on a specific form that is dated and signed by the client, should the nurse waive confidentiality. The client must also be competent to make such a decision. In the event a client is obviously unable to make an informed decision or has been legally declared incompetent, the nurse must implement measures that reflect local, state, and federal regulations to ensure confidentiality. Clients are considered competent unless the client's behavior calls it into question (e.g., strange or aberrant behavior) (Barloon, 2003).

In the case of a minor, a parent or legal guardian has the right to consent for treatment based on age, the nature of the child's diagnosis, or other considerations delineated by state or federal law (American Academy of Pediatrics, 1999). Adolescents may be concerned about confidentiality when sharing information with the nurse. It is imperative to reassure the youth that information shared with his or her parents will be limited by the contents of his or her signed consent form, except in circumstances involving danger to self or others. Some jurisdictions make an exception for adolescents to consent for treatment of substance use disorders, including prescribing contraceptives and treating sexually transmitted diseases, allowing maintenance of confidentiality between the youth and nurse (Muscari, 1998; National Clearinghouse for Alcohol and Drug Information [NCADI]). Federal regulations permit disclosure without the adolescent's consent in several situations, including medical emergencies, reporting child abuse, and communications among health care providers. Nurses must be cognizant of local regulations and statutes and federal regulations that address privacy and confidentiality issues. Family circumstances; the nature, severity, and complexity of the adolescent's problems; age; and emotional, cognitive, and social maturity must also be considered when issues concerning confidentiality exist.

Efforts to maintain confidentiality are important; however, certain circumstances may make it necessary to share information with others, particularly when a person's life or safety are at risk. The duty to protect life often outweighs the duty for confidentiality. Clearly the issues of confidentiality challenge nurses on a daily basis (see Research Study 1-1 on page 44).

CRITICAL THINKING QUESTION

During an interview with a 15-year-old adolescent at a high school health fair, he mentions that he wants to discuss something with you, but you must promise not to share it with his parents. What is the most appropriate response?

1. Make the promise and *only* share it if warranted due to threats to harm himself or others.

2. Inform him that his permission will be requested before specific information is shared with parents, except in situations that involve danger to himself or others.

3. Ask his parents to come into the room so you are not caught in the middle of the youth's and parents' problems.

4. Let him know that his parents have a right to read his record because he is a minor.

Information Technology and Security

Increasingly, identifiable personal information about clients and general health care data are available in electronic form in health databases and online servers. Although access to this information benefits clients and health care providers, enhances client autonomy, improves treatment outcomes, and advances health research, it also has the potential to jeopardize client rights and confidentiality and heightens the risk of abuse or use of information other than for medical purposes.

Technologies have the capacity to transform communication between nurses and their clients and nursing care (Phillips, 2005). Electronic health records and health information can be obtained from handheld computers. A handheld computer is an example of a technology that can help nurses to access electronic progress notes, laboratory and diagnostic results, and orders, which are important communication venues that improve nursing care to clients (Thompson, 2005). Cell phones and pagers can be used to communicate with clients and their families in emergency departments, busy urgent clinic and ambulatory care settings concerning when they will be seen. During these waiting periods, clients and families have the option of getting a meal or staying in the waiting area.

As previously mentioned the spectrum and technologies, including telemedicine, provide vast opportunities for the nurse to communicate and work with clients and families in their homes and communities. Frequently, telemedicine is welcomed by clients who live in rural areas or urban areas in which the client with comorbid chronic diseases is dependent on public transportation. It provides contact with clients who are isolated from their families; psychoeducation about disease management; and emotional support through telehealth monitoring devices and telephonic follow-up.

Documentation

Based on legal and ethical principles, documentation of written communication must be accurate, completed in a timely manner, succinct, unbiased, based on a comprehensive and accurate assessment, and provide evidence to support observations and interpretations (Mohr, 1999). It must also be evidence-based, and reflect professional practice standards and state and federal regulations.

Nowadays documentation is the basis of reimbursement for health care. Numerous agencies depend upon accurate and timely written communication.

Duty to Protect Third Parties

When is it okay to waive the client confidentiality without written consent? There may be several answers to this query, but the most important is when a client threatens to seriously harm or kill a third party or when the nurse suspects child or elder abuse and neglect.

In the first situation, the courts have found that the duty to protect the public, designated as the "duty to warn" or "duty to inform," outweighs the nurse's obligation of confidentiality to the client. The landmark decision that provides the basis of the duty to warn was established by the California Supreme Court in *Tarasoff v. Regents of University of California* (1974), in which the court proclaimed that the privilege of confidentiality ceases when danger to the public exists. Health care providers are protected against breach of confidentiality when the warning is in good faith (Walcott, Cerundolo, & Beck, 2001). The debate over this issue continues, and many feel it threatens the integrity of the nurse–client relationship, particularly in the area of trust. However, clients of nurse psychotherapists, who are routinely informed of the limitations of confidentiality, have little difficulty dealing with this issue. It is imperative that the decision to warn be evaluated individually and based on sound clinical judgment, professional responsibility, and state and federal regulations and laws.

In the second situation, when there is suspicion of child or elder abuse or neglect, all states have mandatory reporting laws for health care providers. The decision to report abuse or neglect in these populations must be based on clear evidence of abuse or neglect and astute clinical judgment. It is imperative for the nurse to be cognizant of reporting regulations and report the abuse in a timely manner and in good faith.

Professional Boundaries

Maintaining **professional boundaries** between the nurse and client is an important ethical and legal issue that is often overlooked. Why are professional boundaries important? Professional boundaries are essential because they define who participates in the interpersonal relationship, nature of relationship, role expectations in the interpersonal relationship, and protect the separateness of the nurse–client relationship.

Boundaries, like space, are defined by numerous factors including culture, ethnicity, stress and anxiety levels, and the ability to form healthy interactions. Persons with certain psychiatric conditions, such as personality disorders, have difficulty discerning boundaries and are likely to test limits by stepping over boundaries. The client will often be excessively clingy and smothering. The inability to form healthy boundaries stems from early childhood relationships that made it difficult to emotionally separate from others and maintain healthy interpersonal boundaries. In these situations it is imperative for the nurse to recognize, develop, and maintain consistent and distinct boundaries between themselves and their clients (see Table 1-3). In contrast, clients with schizophrenia have difficulty feeling close to others and tend to have distant relationships with others. It is imperative to value the need for distance and to create environments that reduce anxiety and tension and the risk of becoming dangerous due to a need to protect self. The client's level of dangerousness is likely to increase when the nurse gets into her or his personal space or touches or makes sudden movements toward clients who prefer aloofness or distant boundaries.

In conclusion, the following strategies can facilitate clear boundaries:

- Be self-aware about your own family systems and clarity regarding the boundaries between self and others and how they continue to influence personal and professional interactions, such as with colleagues and clients.
- Learn to speak for yourself and not others and vice versa.
- Think in terms of what you want and need rather than what others want/need.

Table 1-3 Strategies that Facilitate Professional Boundaries

- Clearly delineated rules that describe who participates and how
- Articulated rules and roles in relationships
- Protected separateness in nurse–client relationship
- Balanced intellectual and emotional systems
- Healthy interpersonal and communication skills
- Recognition and value of cultural factors (both the nurse's and client's), which define boundaries between the nurse and client

- Use "I" statements and take responsibility for the way you feel, think, and behave.
- Afford yourself and others privacy and opportunities or tasks that foster differentiation or self-growth.
- Celebrate your attributes or differences in relationships—both personal and professional.
- Seek opportunities for personal growth and successes.
- Establish and maintain clear boundaries between self and others, recognizing your needs and those of others.
- Avoid taking responsibility for others' feelings, thoughts, and behaviors.
- Avoid speaking for others or propose to know what they are feeling or thinking.

For more information on this topic, see Chapter 5, Professional Development: Leading Through Effective Communication.

SUMMARY

Clearly, communication is important for survival, expressing feelings, imparting information, and working with others to develop treatment approaches that address the needs of clients, families, colleagues, and stakeholders. However, it is imperative for students, novices, and experienced nurses to understand the complexity and difficulty of being effective communicators. Because of daily interactions with clients and staff, the nurse must deal with each encounter individually because what constitutes effective communication in one situation may be ineffective in another (Zoppi & Epstein, 2002).

Communication is a complex and dynamic interaction that requires active listening skills, personal insight or self-awareness, mindfulness, and the appropriate expression of feelings and anxiety. Nurses must identify their communication patterns and styles and understand their impact on relationships with others. The focal point of this chapter has been communication across the life span and the role of diverse and complex factors that enhance or impede effective communication. Despite the difficulty, nurses must be competent and effective communicators. Effective communication skills are necessary to establish interpersonal relationships with physicians and other staff, clients, and their families; these relationships are essential in today's fast-paced, information-driven society and health care arena. Collectively, these factors may enhance client adherence, increase staff and client satisfaction, and facilitate positive clinical outcomes.

SUGGESTIONS FOR CLINICAL AND EXPERIENTIAL ACTIVITIES

1. Use a clinical situation and role play interactions between the nurse and a difficult client. Ask the group to critique and provide constructive feedback.
2. Role-play various types of body language (nonverbal communication) and ask participants to discuss their interpretation and how accurate they are.
3. Provide several scenarios that address life span issues including how to respond to:
   a. An adolescent who asks for reassurance that information shared remains confidential
   b. An older adult with cognitive deficits
4. Ask a nurse or other staff member to discuss nurse–physician issues along with strategies used to resolve workplace conflicts and work effectively as a team to ensure quality health care.

END-OF-CHAPTER QUESTIONS

1. Mr. Johnson, a 79-year-old, is upset because his wife has recently been diagnosed with Alzheimer's disease. He yells at you and calls you "stupid." What is the most appropriate response?
   a. Raise your voice slightly and let him know how it feels when this occurs.
   b. Maintain your composure and let him yell.
   c. Let him know you understand he is upset, but it's difficult to assist when he yells.
   d. Report him to security.
2. Mary is a 35-year-old physician recently diagnosed with Crohn's disease. She is openly upset, yet expresses concerns about her illness and treatment options. She talks to her spouse, who is very supportive. Based on your understanding of attachment styles, which one does Mary exhibit?
   a. Insecure
   b. Secure
   c. Adaptive
   d. Maladaptive
3. Peplau's interpersonal theory discusses four phases of the nurse–client relationship. Which of the following *best* exemplifies the exploitation phase?
   a. Encourage the client to seek guidance in decision making.
   b. Ask the client to identify and discuss personal needs and preferences.

   c. Communicate with significant others about the client's condition.

   d. Tell the client that you are available if he needs your help.

4. Sonny, the evening nurse, is upset about his client's recent diagnosis of a terminal illness. He reports that he has been unable to sleep the past few days because the client reminds him of his father. He also finds himself overly involved in the client's care. Which of the following *best* describes the nurse's behavior?

   a. Unclear boundaries

   b. Empathy

   c. Sympathy

   d. Disclosure

5. Mr. Morris, a new client in the ambulatory care clinic, is very distrustful and refuses to share information with the nurse. Which of the following is the *most* appropriate approach or response to the client?

   a. Avoid talking to him until he is more cooperative.

   b. Review his record for additional information.

   c. Refer him to a mental health professional.

   d. Ask a colleague to talk to him.

6. Which of the following has the greatest impact on communication with adolescents?

   a. Concerns about confidentiality

   b. Overly sensitive to criticism

   c. Poor impulse control

   d. All of the above

7. Mrs. Smyth, an 81-year-old, has an appointment in the primary care clinic. Based on your understanding about communicating with older adults, what is the *least* effective approach to facilitating the nurse–client relationship?

   a. "Mrs. Smyth, I will speak loud so you can hear me."

   b. "How can I help you today?"

   c. "I noticed this is your first visit to the clinic."

   d. "What's brought you in today?"

8. During an interview with Jasmine, a 17-year-old, she asks you to promise not to tell her parents she is taking birth control pills. What is the *most* appropriate response?

   a. "Everything you share is confidential and will not be shared with your parents."

   b. "Jasmine, I am unwilling to keep a secret from your parents."

   c. "Let's bring your parents in so you can share the secret with them, too."

   d. "Jasmine, information about birth control pills will not be shared with your parents."

Answers

8. d
7. a
6. d
5. b
4. c
3. b
2. b
1. c

Research Study 1–1

Title: Disclosing Genetic Test Results to Family Members Hamilton, R. J., Bowers, B. J., & Williams, J. K. (2005). *Journal of Nursing Scholarship, 37,* 18–24.

Purpose: To describe the experiences of disclosing genetic test results to biological family members of people tested for Huntington's disease or hereditary diseases (e.g., cancers).

Design: Grounded theory technology.

Methods: Researchers used open-ended interviews with $n = 29$ participants, of whom 24 had received genetic tests and 5 had not been tested. Population was from 3 countries, including 15 participants from the United States. Interviews were conducted over a 2-month to 4-year period. Taped interviews were transcribed and analyzed for conceptual categorization to depict personal meanings of disclosing test results.

Results/Findings: Participants described the impact of disclosing test results to family members and how they selectively made decisions to disclose. Timing of the disclosure was impacted by the nature of the disease and the participant's personal need to prepare. Disclosure brought about genetic risk or disease-generated discussion between the participant and family member.

Implications for Nurses: Various legal and ethical issues guide disclosure of genetic diseases and risk. The decision to share genetic test results and other health data with families is based on the individual's consent. Nurses are in key positions to facilitate therapeutic relationships with clients faced with their own issues associated with genetic testing and disclosing them with family members.

REFERENCES

Agency for Healthcare Research and Quality. (2001). *Telemedicine for the Medicare population: Summary.* AHRQ Publication Number 01-E011. Rockville, MD: Agency for Healthcare Research and Quality. Retrieved March 27, 2005, from http://text.nlm.nih.gov/ftrs/directBrowse.pl?collect=epc&dbname=telesum

Ainsworth, M. S., Blehar, M. C., Waters, E., & Wall, S. (1978). *Patterns of attachment: A psychological study of the strange situation.* Hillsdale, NJ: Erlbaum Associates.

Alberca, R., Montes, E., Russell, E., Gil-Néciga, E., & Mesulam, M. (2004). Left hemicranial hypoplasia in 2 patients with primary progressive aphasia. *Archives of Neurology, 61,* 265–268.

American Academy of Pediatrics. (1999). Privacy protection of health information: Patient rights and pediatrician responsibilities. *Pediatrics, 104,* 973–977. Retrieved May 13, 2005, from http://aappolicy.aappublications.org/cgi/reprint/pediatrics; 104/4/973.pdf

American Nurses Association. (2001). *Code of ethics for nurses with interpretative statements.* Washington, DC: Author.

American Psychiatric Association. (2000). *Diagnostic and statistical manual of mental disorders* (4th ed., text rev.). Washington, DC: Author.

Amini, F., Lewis, T., Lannon, R., Louie, A., Baumbacher, G., McGuinness, T., et al. (1996). Affect, attachment, memory: Contributions toward psychobiologic integration. *Psychiatry, 59,* 213–239.

Antai-Otong, D. (2002). Culturally sensitive treatment of African Americans with substance-related disorders. *Journal of Psychosocial Nursing and Mental Health Services, 40,* 14–21.

Antai-Otong, D., & Wasserman, F. (2003). Therapeutic communication. In D. Antai-Otong (ed.), *Psychiatric Nursing: Biological and Behavioral Concepts* (pp. 127–150). Clifton Park, NY: Delmar Thomson Learning.

Barloon, L. F. (2003). Legal aspects of psychiatric nursing, *The Nursing Clinics of North America, 38,* 9–19.

Barrick, T. R., Mackay, C. E., Prima, S., Maes, F., Vandermeulen, D., Crow, T. J., et al. (2005). Automatic analysis of cerebral symmetry: An exploratory study of the relationship between brain torque and planum temporale asymmetry. *Neuroimaging, 24,* 678–691.

Bartholomew, K. (1990). Avoidance of intimacy: An attachment perspective. *Journal of Social and Personal Relationships, 7,* 147–178.

Bartholomew, K. (1993). From childhood to adult relationships: Attachment theory and research. In S. Duck (ed.), *Learning About Relationships: Understanding Relationships Processes Series* (vol. 2, pp. 30–63). Newbury Park, CA: Sage.

Bartholomew, K., & Horowitz, L. M. (1991). Attachment styles among young adults: A test of a four-category model. *Journal of Personality and Social Psychology, 61,* 226–244.

Berger, J. T. (1998). Culture and ethnicity in clinical care. *Archives of Internal Medicine, 158,* 2085–2090.

Berlo, D. K. (1960). *The process of communication: An introduction to theory and practice.* New York: Holt, Rinehart, Winston.

Bernstein, P. S., Farinelli, C., & Merkatz, I. R. (2005). Using an electronic medical record to improve communication within a prenatal care network. *Obstetrics and Gynecology, 105,* 607–612.

Boise, L., & White, D. (2004). The family's role in person-centered care: Practice considerations. *Journal of Psychosocial Nursing and Mental Health Services, 42,* 12–20.

Bowlby, J. (1969). *Attachment and loss* (Vol. 1). New York: Basic Books.

Bowlby, J. (1973). *Attachment and loss* (Vol. 2). New York: Basic Books.

Bowlby, J. (1980). *Attachment and loss* (Vol. 3). New York: Basic Books.

Boyle, D. K., & Kochinda, C. (2004). Enhancing collaborative communication of nurse and physician leadership in two intensive care units. *The Journal of Nursing Administration, 34,* 60–70.

Brennan, K. A., & Shaver, P. R. (1998). Attachment styles and personality disorders: Their connections to each other and to parental divorce, parental death, and perceptions of parental caregiving. *Journal of Personality, 66,* 835–878.

Brown, J. B., Boles, M., Mullooly, J. P., & Levinson, W. (1999). Effect of clinician communication skills training on patient satisfaction. *Annals of Internal Medicine, 131,* 822–829.

Buschsbaum, M. S. (2004). Frontal lobe function. Images in neuroscience. *American Journal of Psychiatry, 162,* 2178.

Ceccio, J. F., & Ceccio, C. M. (1982). *Effective communication in nursing: Theory and practice.* New York: John Wiley & Sons.

Christensen, A., & Frank-Stromborg, M. (2001). The protection of patient privacy in a high-tech era. *Journal of Nursing Law, 8,* 17–21.

Cioffi, R. N. (2003). Communicating with culturally and linguistically diverse patients in an acute care setting: Nurses' experiences. *International Journal of Nursing Studies, 40,* 299–306.

Colins, N. L., & Feeney, B. C. (2000). A safe haven: An attachment theory perspective on support seeking and caregiving in intimate relationships. *Journal of Personality and Social Psychology, 78,* 1053–1073.

Cooper-Patrick, L., Gallo, J. J., Gonzales, J. J., et al. (1999). Race, gender, and partnership in the patient-physician relationship. *Journal of the American Medical Association, 282,* 583–589.

David, A. S. (1999). Auditory hallucinations: Phenomenology, neuropsychology and neuroimaging update. *Acta Psychiatrica Scandinavia Supplement, 395,* 95–104.

Duffy, F. D., Gordon, G. H., Whelan, G., Cole-Kelly, K., Frankel, R., Buffone, N., et al. (2004). Participants in the American Academy on Physician and Patient's Conference on Education and Evaluation of Competence in Communication and Inter-personal Skills. *Academy of Medicine, 79,* 495–507.

Einbinder, L. C., & Schulman, K. A. (2000). The effect of race on the referral process for invasive cardiac procedures. *Medical Care Research Review, 1,* 162–177.

Erikson, E. H. (1963). *Childhood and society.* New York: W. W. Norton.

Faroqi-Shah, Y., & Thompson, C. K. (2003). Effect of lexical cues on the production of active and passive sentences in Broca and Wernicke's aphasia. *Brain Language, 85,* 409–426.

Fernald, A., Swingley, D., & Pinto, J. P. (2001). Cognition and language: When half a word is enough: Infants can recognize spoken words during partial phonetic infor-mation. *Child Development, 72,* 1003–1015.

Flagg, E. J., Cardy, J. E., Roberts, W., & Roberts, T. P. (2005). Language lateralization development in children with autism. *Neuroscience Letter, 386,* 82–87.

Flores, G. (2000). Culture and the patient-physician relationship: Achieving cultural competency in health care. *Journal of Pediatrics, 136,* 14–23.

Foundas, A. L., Leonard, C. M., Gilmore, R., Fennell, E., & Heilman, K. M. (1996). Pars triangularis asymmetry and language dominance. *Proceedings of the National Academy of Science, 93,* 719–722.

Frank, E. M. (1994). Effect of Alzheimer's disease on communication function. *The Journal of South Carolina Medical Association, 90,* 417–423.

Furr, R. M., & Funder, D. C. (1998). A multimodal analysis of personal negativity. *Journal of Personality and Social Psychology, 74,* 1580–1591.

Ganong, W. F. (1999). *Review of medical physiology* (19th ed.). Stamford, CT: Appleton & Lange.

Goldberg, D. (2003). Vulnerability, destabilization and restitution in anxious depres-sion. *Acta Psychiatrica Scandinavia, 108*(Suppl. 418), 81–82.

Hall, E. T. (1966). *The hidden dimension.* Garden City, NJ: Doubleday.

Hall, E. T. (1989). *Beyond culture.* New York: Doubleday.

Harms, C., Young, J. R., Amsler, F., Zettler, C., Scheidegger, D., & Kindler, C. H. (2004). Improving anesthetists' communication skills. *Anaesthesia, 59,* 166–172.

Howells, J. G. (1975). *Principles of family psychotherapy.* New York: Brunnel/ Mazel.

Hubl, D., Koenig, T., Strik, W., Federepiel, A., Kreis, R., Boesch, C., et al. (2004). Pathways that make voices. *Archives of General Psychiatry, 61,* 658–668.

Kagawa-Singer, M., & Kassim-Lakha, S. (2003). A strategy to reduce cross-cultural miscommunication and increase the likelihood of improving health outcomes. *Aca-demic Medicine, 78,* 577–587.

Kavanagh, K. H., & Kennedy, P. H. (1992). *Promoting cultural diversity.* Newbury Park, CA: Sage.

Keltner, D., & Haidt, J. (2001). Social functions of emotions. In T. J. May & G. A. Bonnano (eds.), *Emotions: Current Issues and Future Directions. Emotions and Social Behavior* (pp. 192–213). New York: Guilford Press.

Kidd, T., & Sheffield, D. (2005). Attachment style and symptom reporting: Examining the mediating effects of anger and social support. *British Journal of Health and Psychology, 10,* 531–541.

Kimura, D. (1983). Speech representation in an unbiased sample of left-handers. *Human Neurobiology, 2,* 142–154.

Kleinman, A., Eisenberg, L., & Good, B. (1978). Culture, illness and care: Clinical lessons from anthropologic and cross-cultural research. *Annals of Internal Medicine, 88,* 251–258.

Kleinman, S. (2004). What is the nature of nurse practitioners' lived experiences interacting with patients? *Journal of the American Academy of Nurse Practitioners, 16,* 263–269.

Klin, A., Jones, W., Schutlz, R., Volkmar, F., & Cohen, D. (2002). Defining and qualifying the social phenotype in autism. *American Journal of Psychiatry, 159,* 895–908.

Larson, E. (1999). The impact of physician-nurse interaction on patient care. *Holistic Nursing Practice, 13,* 38–46.

Leininger, M. (2002). Culture care theory: A major contribution to advance transcultural nursing knowledge and practices. *Journal of Transcultural Nursing, 13,* 189–192.

Levinson, W., & Chaumeton, N. (1999). Communication between surgeons and patients in routine office visits. *Surgery, 125,* 127–134.

Levitan, S., Ward, P. B., & Catts, S. V. (1999). Superior temporal gyral volumes and laterality correlates of auditory hallucinations in schizophrenia. *Biological Psychiatry, 46,* 955–962.

Mayhew, P. A., Acton, G. J., Yauk, S., & Hopkins, B. A. (2001). Communication from individuals with advanced DAT: Can it provide clues to their sense of self-awareness and well-being. *Geriatric Nursing, 22,* 106–110.

Mesulam, M. M. (1990). Large-scale neurocognitive networks and distributed processes for attention, language, and memory. *Annals of Neurology, 28,* 597–613.

Mohr, W. K. (1999). Deconstructing the language of psychiatric hospitalization. *Journal of Advanced Nursing, 29,* 1052–1059.

Moore, T. F., & Hollett, J. (2003). Giving voice to persons with dementia: The researcher's opportunities and challenges. *Nursing Science Quarterly, 16,* 163–167.

Munet-Vilaró, F. (2004). Delivery of culturally competent care to children with cancer and their families—The Latino experience. *Journal of Pediatric Oncology Nursing, 21,* 155–159.

Murray-Garcia, J. L., Selby, J. V., Schmittdiehl, J., Grumbach, K., & Quesenberry, C. P. (2000). Racial and ethnic differences in patient survey: Patients' values ratings and reports regarding physician primary care performance in a large health maintenance organization. *Medical Care, 38,* 300–310.

Muscari, M. E. (1998). When can an adolescent give consent? *American Journal of Nursing, 98,* 18–19.

National Clearinghouse for Alcohol and Drug Information (NCADI). Treatment of adolescents with substance use disorders treatment improvement protocol (TIP);

Series 32. Chapter 8—Legal and ethical issues. Retrieved May 18, 2005, from http://www.health.org/govpubs/ bkd307/32k.aspx

National Research Council. (2000). *Networking health: Prescriptions for the Internet.* Washington, DC: National Academy Press.

Noterdaeme, M., Mildenberger, K., Minow, F., & Amorosa, H. (2002). Evaluation of neuromotor deficits in children with autism and children with a specific speech and language disorder. *European Children and Adolescent Psychiatry, 11,* 219–225.

Office of Minority Health. (2001). Culturally and linguistically appropriate services. Retrieved May 6, 2005, from http://www.omhrc.gov/CLAS/finalcultural1a.htm

Ognibene, T. C., & Collins, N. L. (1998). Adult attachment styles, perceived social support and coping strategies. *Journal of Social and Personality Relationships, 15,* 323–345.

Papazissis, E. (2004). Advanced technology permits the provision of advanced hospital care in the patients' homes. *Studies of Health Technology and Information, 100,* 190–199.

Peplau, H. E. (1952). *Interpersonal relations in nursing.* New York: G. P. Putnam's Sons.

Peplau, H. E. (1991/1952). *Interpersonal relations in nursing: A conceptual frame of reference for psychodynamic nursing.* New York: Springer.

Phillips, J. (2005). Knowledge is power: Using nursing information management and leadership interventions to improve services to patients, clients and users. *Journal of Nursing Management, 13,* 524–536.

Prather, P. A., Zurif, E., Love, T., & Brownell, H. (1997). Speech of lexical activation in nonfluent Broca's aphasia and fluent Wernicke's aphasia. *Brain Language, 59,* 391–411.

Pugh, K. R., Mencl, W. E., Jenner, A. R., Katz, L., Frost, S. J., Lee, J. R., et al. (2001). Neurological studies of reading and reading disability. *Communication Disorders, 34,* 479–492.

Rogers, C. (1974). *Carl Rogers on personal power.* New York: Delacorte Press.

Rosenstein, A. H. (2002). Original research: Nurse-physician relationships: Impact on nurse satisfaction and retention. *American Journal of Nursing, 102,* 26–34.

Rosenstein, A. H., & O'Daniel, M. (2005). Disruptive behavior and clinical outcomes: Perceptions of nurses and physicians. *American Journal of Nursing, 105,* 54–64.

Roter, D. L., Stewart, M., Putnam, S. M., Lipkin, M. Jr, Stiles, W., & Inui, T. S. (1997). Communication patterns of primary care physicians. *Journal of the American Medical Association, 277,* 350–356.

Rutter, M. (2000). Genetic studies of autism: From the 1970's into the millennium. *Journal of Abnormal Psychology, 28,* 3–14.

Satir, V. (1967). *Conjoint family therapy* (rev. ed.). Palo Alto, CA: Science and Behavior Books.

Schmidt, I. K., & Svarstad, B. L. (2002). Nurse-physician communication and quality of drug use in Swedish nursing homes. *Sociology Science Medicine, 54,* 1767–1777.

Schore, A. N. (1997). Early organization of the nonlinear right brain and development of predisposition to psychiatric disorders. *Developmental Psychopathology, 9,* 595–631.

Schore, A. N. (2000). Attachment and the regulation of the right brain. *Attachment and Human Behavior, 2,* 23–47.

Schore, A. N. (2001). Effects of secure attachment relationship on right brain development, affect regulation, and infant mental health. *Infant Mental Health Journal, 22,* 7–66.

Schwartz, E. R. (1990). Speech and language disorders. In M. W. Schwartz (ed.), *Pediatric Primary Care: A Problem-Oriented Approach* (pp. 696–700). St. Louis, MO: Mosby.

Segalowitz, S. J., & Bryden, M. P. (1983). Individual differences in hemispheric representation of language. In S. J. Segalowitz (ed.), *Language and Brain Organization* (pp. 341–372). New York: Academic Press.

Shaywitz, S. E., Shaywitz, B. A., Fulbright, R. K., Skudlarski, P., Mencl, W. E., Constable, R. T., et al. (2003). Neural systems for compensation and persistence: Young adult outcome of childhood reading disability. *Biological Psychiatry, 54,* 25–33.

Sheldon, B. (1994). Communicating with Alzheimer's patients. *Journal of Gerontological Nursing, 20,* 51–53.

Shulman, M. D., & Mandel, E. (1993). Maximizing communication with the Alzheimer's patient. *Nursing Home, 9,* 36–38.

Simos, P. G., Breier, J. I., Fletcher, J. M., Bergman, E., & Papanicolaou, A. C. (2000). Cerebral mechanisms involved in word reading in dyslexic children: A magnetic resonance imaging approach. *Cerebral Cortex, 10,* 809–816.

Sinha, R., Lacadie, C., Skudarski, P., & Wexler, B. E. (2004). Neural circuits underlying emotional distress in humans. *Annals of New York Academy of Science, 1032,* 254–257.

Slade, P., & Bentall, R. (2002). *Sensory deception: A scientific analysis of hallucination.* London: Croom Helm.

Sloan, D. M., Bradley, M. M., Dinoulas, E., & Lang, P. J. (2002). Looking at facial expression: Dysphoria and facial EMG. *Biological Psychiatry, 60,* 79–90.

Smith, C. A., & Pope, L. K. (1992). Appraisal and emotion: The interactional contributions of dispositional and situational factors. In M. S. Clark (Ed.), *Review of Personality and Social Psychology* (Vol. 14, pp. 32–62). Newbury Park, CA: Sage.

Street, R. L. Jr. (2002). Gender differences in health care provider-patient communication: Are they due to style, stereotypes, or accommodation? *Patient Education Counseling, 48,* 201–206.

Taira, D. A., Sarfan, D. G., Seto, T. B., et al. (1997). Asian-American patient ratings of physician primary care performance. *Journal of General Internal Medicine, 12,* 237–242.

Tappen, R. M., Williams, C., Fishman, S., & Touhy, T. (1999). Persistence of self in advanced Alzheimer's disease. *Image Journal of Nursing Scholarship, 31,* 121–125.

Tappen, R. M., Williams-Burgess, C., Edelstein, J., Touhy, T., & Fishman, S. (1997). Communicating with individuals with Alzheimer's disease: An examination of recommended strategies. *Archives of Psychiatric Nursing, 9,* 249–256.

Tarasoff v. Regents of University of California, 118 California Reported 129, 529 P. 2d 553 (Supreme Court 1974).

Thompson, B. W. (2005). The transforming effect of handheld computers on nursing practice. *Nursing Admininstration Quarterly, 29,* 308–314.

U.S. Census Bureau. (2000). U.S. Census. Retrieved March 1, 2005, from http://www.census.gov

U.S. Department of Health and Human Services. (1992). *Cultural competence for evaluators: A guide for alcohol and other drug abuse prevention practitioners working with ethnic/racial communities.* Rockville, MD: Author.

Van Ryn, M., & Burke, J. (2000). The effect of patient race and socio-economic status on physician's perception of patients. *Social Science Medicine, 50,* 813–828.

Walcott, D. M., Cerundolo, P., & Beck, J. C. (2001). Current analysis of the Tarasokk duty: An evolution towards limitation of the duty to protect. *Behavioral Science Law, 10,* 325–343.

Waters, E., & Cummings, E. M. (2000). A secure base from which to explore close relationships. *Child Development, 71,* 164–172.

Webster's New Collegiate Dictionary (1974). Springfield. MA: G & C Merriam Company.

Weisbrot, D. M., & Carlson, G. A. (2005). Is it ADHD? Mania? Autism? What to do if no diagnosis fits. *Current Psychiatry, 4,* 25–28, 35–36, 39–40, 42.

West, M., Rose, M. S., Verhoff, M. J., Spreng, S., & Bobey, M. (1998). Anxious attachment and self-reported depressive symptomatology in women. *Canadian Journal of Psychiatry, 43,* 294–297.

Winn, P., Cook, J. B., & Bonnel, W. (2004). Improving communication among attending physicians, long-term care facilities, residents and residents' families. *American Medical Directors Association, 5,* 114–122.

Zoppi, K., & Epstein, R. M. (2002). Is communication a skill? Communication behaviors and being in relation. *Family Medicine, 35,* 310–324.

SELECTED WEB SITES

Access Project (Limited English project): http://www.accessproject.org

Autism Spectrum Disorders (Pervasive Developmental Disorders): http://www.nimh.nih.gov/healthinformation/autismmenu.cfm

National Institute of Mental Health Outreach:
http://www.nimh.nih.gov/outreach/index.cfm

National Institute on Deafness and Other Communication Disorders:
http://www.nidcd.nih.gov

Office for Civil Rights: http://www.hhs.gov/ocr/hipaa/finalmaster.html

Chapter Two

Therapeutic Communication Techniques

LEARNING OBJECTIVES

Upon completion of this chapter, the reader should be able to:

- Discuss therapeutic communication techniques
- Analyze barriers that compromise active listening
- Review the impact of culture on nurse–client relationships
- Describe negotiation and conflict management
- Contrast assertive, passive, and aggressive communication skills
- Discuss appropriate use of self-disclosure
- Appraise therapeutic communication techniques across the life span

KEY TERMS

Active listening—An active, selective attentiveness and interactive process that involves all senses, comprehension, and mindfulness to assess verbal and nonverbal communication.

Assertiveness—In communication, this is the process of clearly and confidently expressing one's opinions, needs, wishes, and desires without purposely infringing on the rights of others.

Clarification—A useful technique that helps the nurse validate verbal and nonverbal communication to determine its accuracy.

Conflict—An interpersonal and/or mental struggle arising from opposing demands or impulses. It has the propensity to generate strong feelings, discord, and disagreement.

Conflict resolution—The ability to use assertive communication skills to generate options to effectively resolve disagreements, stress, and turmoil.

Confrontation—A therapeutic technique used to point out incongruence between what is said and one's behavior.

Focusing—Clarifying or validating a perception or understanding of a specific aspect of communication.

Humor—Refers to being amusing, funny, or comical to express feelings and thoughts in a manner comfortable to oneself and others.

Imparting information—Making facts or information available when an individual requests them.

Negotiation—A process or means for achieving a common goal or understanding of what one wants from others. It is a give-and-take communication method designed to obtain an agreement.

Nonverbal communication—"Body language" or expression through movement or behaviors. Examples of body language include physical or behavioral gestures, head nods, eye contact, writing, symbols and pictures, laughter, tone of voice, and facial expressions.

Questioning—The act of asking questions for the purpose of clarifying the meaning of a communication or to collect facts, facilitate feedback, and validate assumptions or perceptions of the sender.

Rapport—A mutually comfortable relationship based on respect, objectivity, trust, and safety. It facilitates communication and is the basis of therapeutic interactions.

Reflection—Restating or paraphrasing and validating what is communicated within a support environment. Often, words or phrases such as "you" or "It sounds like you *feel* . . ." or "You seem *concerned about* . . ." are used to restate what the nurse gleaned from a client's emotions and statements.

Self-disclosure—To share information about oneself.

Silence—A communication technique that makes it clear that every moment does not require verbal exchange; it allows the client to contemplate, focus, and organize thoughts and feelings.

Summarize—The process of integrating or synthesizing key points of the nurse–client discussion and highlighting progress made toward greater understanding. It facilitates a greater understanding of what was communicated and validates that the nurse has heard the same information as the client conveyed.

Therapeutic communication—A healing or curative nurse–client interaction.

Verbalizing the implied—Clarification of what the person hinted at or alluded to, allowing a clearer understanding of the message or conversation.

INTRODUCTION

Nurses have long understood the centrality of therapeutic relationships and the significance of effective nurse–client communication. **Therapeutic communication** is the basis of interactive relationships and affords opportunities to establish rapport, understand the client's experiences, formulate individualized or client-centered interventions, and optimize health care resources. **Rapport** is a mutually comfortable relationship between the nurse and client based on trust and safety. After rapport has been developed, therapeutic interactions allow clients to express feelings and communicate thoughts and uncertainties within an accepting, safe, and supportive environment. Acceptance is not synonymous with agreement or approval; instead, it means understanding and respecting the client's perspective without judging or blaming. The quality of these interactions and the ability to improve on them are frequently governed by diverse factors including the nurse's attitude, his or her ability to understand behavior within a social context, and his or her openness to listening and responding empathetically to others.

Research indicates that quality communication among the client, health care providers, families, and other stakeholders can improve health care and help clients adapt to illness and adhere to interventions. Therapeutic communication, which refers to a healing or curative nurse–client interaction, allays stress in the nurse and client, particularly when they collaborate in the decision-making process for serious or life-threatening issues and informed consent (Lobb, Nutow, Kenny, & Tattersall, 1999; von Gunten, Ferris, & Emanuel, 2000). Failure to convey empathy, calmness, genuine interest, and openness increases anxiety, threatens hope and motivation, impairs decision-making skills, and compromises clinical outcomes (Cooper et al., 2003; Institute of Medicine [IOM], 2001).

Culture and ethnicity also influence the client's perception and expression of anxiety, depression, stress, and participation in treatment planning. Researchers believe that nurse–client interactions must be individualized and adapted to accept diverse modes of communicating the client's experience (Bates, Rankin-Hill, & Sanchez-Ayendez, 1997; Koch, Marks, & Tooke, 2001). Assessing individual differences, personal options, wishes, values, beliefs, and health practices are essential aspects of shared decision making and client-centered care. Embracing individual client needs enables the nurse to form and maintain healing interactions and achieve positive clinical outcomes. In-depth discussions of factors associated with effective communication are discussed in Chapter 1.

Therapeutic communication extends beyond the nurse–client relationship and involves interactions with staff, families, and stakeholders. Stakeholders include individuals or organizations with a vested interested in health care issues and policies, such as communities, higher learning and teaching institutions, government officials, advocacy groups, and financial supporters.

Communication is particularly significant in today's fast-paced, information-driven society because care can become fragmented if clients enter multiple sectors of the health care system. Poor communication among staff creates gaps in the continuity of care and threatens client safety. Gaps or insufficient information sharing between the nurse and other health care providers frequently result in inaccurate health decisions and poor or late-entry documentation, jeopardize client safety, and increase the risk of litigation and poor health outcomes (Branger, van't Hooft, van der Wooden, Duisterhout, & van Bemmel, 1998; Cook, Render, & Woods, 2000; Gosbee, 1998; The, Hak, Koeter, & van Der Wal, 2000; Van Walraven, Seth, & Laupacis, 2002). Finally, as brokers of health care and as client advocates, nurses must use interpersonal relationships and work with others, including the client and family, to ensure holistic, equitable, and quality health care and to facilitate optimal clinical outcomes across the life span.

Information technology affords vast opportunities to communicate and transmit interventions to clients, families, and health care providers through various modalities, ranging from the Internet, Palm Pilots, email, and video cameras to telephone, teleconferencing, and face-to-face meetings. Regardless of the communication method, confidentiality must be ensured and based on ethics and statutory and federal regulations. Nurses also are challenged to navigate through the matrix of telecommunication technologies and create interactive dialogues to establish rapport, provide and monitor care, and analyze nonverbal and verbal data. As health care transforms from inpatient services to working with people in communities and client homes, technological advances such as telehealth and telemedicine will become the primary venue for health care. These venues already exist, allowing client data to be collected and analyzed using video monitoring, telephone messaging, and other innovative communication devices to advance health care across the continuum of care (Breslin, Greskovich, & Turisco, 2004; Grant, Cagliero, Chuch, & Meigs, 2005). Emerging research indicates that using technology to communicate with the client and family provides positive treatment outcomes such as enhanced self-care management, while also increasing provider and client satisfaction, improving resource allocation, and reducing health care costs (Baker, Rideout, Gertler, & Raube, 2005; Liu, Pothiban, Lu, & Khamphonsiri, 2000).

This chapter focuses on effective communication techniques that can be used in a variety of practice settings. It offers both the novice and experienced nurse a cadre of techniques, such as active listening, assertiveness, conflict resolution, and negotiation, to create a healthy work environment. Collectively, these techniques demonstrate respect for self and others, and provide a powerful foundation to advance and broker client-centered health care across the life span.

THERAPEUTIC COMMUNICATION TECHNIQUES

Therapeutic nurse–client interactions require warmth, trust, empathy, and mutual respect. What's more, the client must believe the nurse cares, understands, and is concerned about his or her problem. A caring and safe environment helps the nurse embrace and value the client's internal and external experience, strengthen shared decision making, elicit relevant clinical data, and formulate individualized care. The following sections discuss these key therapeutic communication techniques:

- Active listening
- Assertiveness
- Clarification
- Conflict resolution
- Confrontation
- Focusing
- Giving or imparting information
- Humor

- Negotiation
- Questioning
- Reflection
- Self-disclosure
- Silence
- Summarizing
- Verbalizing the implied

Active Listening

Everyone loves a good listener, but not everyone is a good listener. **Active listening** is the cornerstone of all interactions. It is difficult to assess the client's needs, wishes, or concerns unless you take time to listen to them. Listening extends beyond the act of hearing words and includes understanding and accurately interpreting what the client *really* says. Listening extends beyond being silent; it is an interactive and dynamic process. Active listening requires the use of all the senses and involves attention, comprehension, and mindfulness to assess verbal and **nonverbal communication**. It requires genuine interest in others' points of view. Through mental processes, we are able to selectively attend to a desired message or communication. This dynamic and interactive process requires vast energy, self-control, patience, genuine interest, and concentration. It also involves establishing a dialogue and encouraging the client to set the tone and become more direct. This may be difficult for clients with low self-esteem or poor interpersonal or social skills, such as those with major mental health problems like schizophrenia, depression, and social phobia, or those with cognitive disturbances (e.g., confusional states). In these situations the nurse must be more directive and provide a structure that enhances nurse–client interactions.

Listening is a faster process than speaking. Communication experts estimate that regardless of how rapidly a person speaks she cannot speak more than 200–250 words per minute. In comparison, the listener can take in words as fast as he thinks. It is very important to pay close attention to the speaker's entire statement and avoid completing sentences or interrupting. Although the nurse has little control over how rapidly the client speaks, it is crucial to maintain self-control and listen attentively to accurately interpret verbal and nonverbal cues. Active listening is an investment in the nurse–client relationship and eventually creates an environment that fosters trust and security and elicits relevant data to make accurate diagnoses, establish shared decision making, implement individualized interventions, and advance positive clinical outcomes.

Ceccio and Ceccio (1982) distinguished the following characteristics of good listening:

- Maintain eye contact.
- Give full attention, both mentally and physically (make a conscious effort to screen or filter distractions; listen from the heart).
- Reduce barriers.
- Avoid interruptions.
- Respond to the content and emotional (feeling) component of the message.
- Listen for ideas or themes.
- Convey evidence of listening (e.g., paraphrasing, restating what is said, or playing back the message).
- Respond to the content and emotional aspect of the client's verbal and nonverbal message.

The nurse must demonstrate active listening while conversing with the client. Evidence of genuine interest and listening is established by eye contact, facial expression, facing the person with an open and relaxed posture, nodding the head to suggest agreement and acknowledgement, leaning forward, and summarizing. Comments such as "It sounds like you are very stressed about losing your job," or "I hear what you are saying and certainly recognize how difficult this is for you" are examples of active listening.

The nurse and client bring a repertoire of personal attributes, life experiences, and ideas about relationships. Active listening challenges the nurse to pay close attention to the client's concerns and communication. Furthermore, the nurse must scrutinize her or his own blinders. Personal scrutiny or self-awareness is an honest and open appraisal of individual filters, culture, and biases that may obscure or distort perceptions and objectivity. Active listening creates a healing climate, which reduces stress and anxiety while expanding self-esteem and adaptive coping behaviors. The quality of a healing climate is determined by self-awareness. The more we know ourselves, the easier it is to objectively listen, tolerate differences, and value others.

Barriers That Compromise Active Listening

It is important to recognize barriers to active listening so they can be addressed and minimized. Interrupting, completing sentences for the speaker, introducing unrelated information, challenging or asking "why" questions, and minimizing feelings deter active listening. Barriers to active listening occur in all settings, and when left unchecked impede effective communication and high-quality interpersonal interactions. Becoming aware of how often you use various barriers is the first step to identifying, reducing, and eventually eliminating them. Review the barriers in Table 2-1 and ask yourself how often you use them. How do others react?

Assertiveness

Assertiveness is the ability to confidently and honestly express your opinions, thoughts, ideas, and rights without undue guilt or anxiety, in a manner that respects personal and others' rights. The primary aim of assertiveness is to meet personal needs and maintain personal rights and respect for self and others. It is a learned behavior, and although it is an important behavior, nurses seldom use it. Regrettably, today's nurses are often reluctant to be assertive. Nurses often have difficulty using assertive communication skills to advance their personal needs and respecting the rights of their nurse col-

Table 2-1 Barriers to Active Listening

- Personal filters: biases, values, beliefs, culture, stereotyping
- High emotional state
- Blaming
- Intimidating body language (e.g., intrusiveness, loud voice, glaring eye contact)
- Hurried approaches
- Closed-mindedness (e.g., all or none thinking, rigidity)
- Using jargon or clichés
- Expressing disapproval (verbal and nonverbal [e.g., raising an eyebrow, frowning])
- Giving advice
- Interrupting
- Asking closed-ended questions
- Minimizing the client's feelings, beliefs, and thoughts
- Showing anxiety or fear
- Language that is different from the clients, such as the client with limited English competency
- Hearing what you want to hear
- Lack of privacy
- Environmental noise
- Sensory or perceptual disturbances
- Cognitive deficits (e.g., age-related, substance abuse)
- Pain in the client

leagues. Influences such as socialization, gender, low self-esteem, low self-confidence, and lack of knowledge frequently underlie this difficulty.

Numerous studies indicate that nurses are unlikely to disagree with others or provide constructive feedback; as a result they experience poor interpersonal relationships with clients and staff, high burnout, loss of autonomy, and job dissatisfaction (McCartan & Hargie, 2004; Timmins & McCabe, 2005a, 2005b). Passiveness produces helplessness, resentment, depression, undue stress, somatic symptoms (e.g., headaches, GI disturbances), frustration, and poor interpersonal relationships and may even cause anger outbursts, violence or aggression, or serious stress-related health problems (Antai-Otong, 2001). Some researchers submit that an answer to this problem may be assertiveness training, which can bolster self-worth, confidence, self-respect, job satisfaction, and interpersonal relationships (Begley & Glacken, 2004; Lin et al., 2004).

Aggressive communication, in contrast, is just as ineffective as passive communication and is frequently used to humiliate, "put down," and embarrass others and eventually destroys interpersonal relationships, reduces productivity, and jeopardizes clinical outcomes (see Table 2-2).

In today's changing health care system, it is vital for nurses to develop and use assertive (not aggressive) communication skills as a means of advancing personal and professional needs, ensuring safe work environments, advocating for quality and holistic health care, and establishing healthy interactions with clients, staff, and various stakeholders. Effective assertive communication skills promote mutual goal setting, team building, and conflict resolution. Successful assertive communication requires recognizing the differences among assertive, passive, and aggressive communication skills and practicing the use of assertiveness rather than passiveness or aggression. The following critical thinking section compares the three skills.

Table 2-2 Comparison of Assertive, Passive, and Aggressive Communication Styles

Assertiveness (win-win position)	Passiveness (lose-win)	Aggressiveness (win-lose)
• "I or me" statements • Respect personal rights and those of others • Confidence • Honesty and appropriate responses • High self-esteem • Risk taker • Says no without undue guilt or anxiety • Direct eye contact • Erect posture • Clear and normal voice tone • Congruent facial expression	• Puts others' needs ahead of own • "Your needs are more important than mine" • Low self-esteem • Highly anxious • Avoids conflicts • "People pleaser" • Permits others to violate rights • Difficulty expressing true or honest feelings • Apologetic • Poor eye contact • Stooped posture • Whiny voice tone • Timid body language • Difficulty saying "no," and when it occurs feels anxious and guilty • Somatic complaints, stress-related physical and mental health problems	• "You" and blaming statements • Meets personal needs with little regards for the rights of others • Loud • Infringes on the rights of others • Intrusive • Glaring eye contact • Intimidating • Embarrassing • Frightening

CRITICAL THINKING QUESTIONS

You are the charge nurse on the midnight shift and one of the medical students approaches you yelling and demanding you to immediately carry out an order just written (a non-STAT order). Prior to being asked to carry out the orders, you discovered a client had slipped in the bathroom and you are helping him.

Question: Which is an assertive response?

Nurse: I understand that you are upset, but it is difficult for me to assist you when you yell, and as you can see we are helping Mr. Jones who just slipped in the bathroom.

Nurse: Yes, Doctor. I am very sorry for not completing the order. Can you wait until I get Mr. Jones out of the bathroom?

Nurse: Now listen! If you want those orders done, do them yourself! Can't you see I'm trying to get Mr. Jones out of the bathroom?

Answer: Obviously, the first response is an assertive response, whereas the second response is passive and the last response is aggressive. The latter two are counterproductive, impede therapeutic interactions, and create new and ongoing problems.

Question: What distinguishes assertive people from passive and aggressive people?

Answer:

Assertive people:
- Are confident
- Respect themselves
- Use "I" or "me" statements rather than "you" statements
- Respect the rights of others
- Clearly speak their point of view
- Take responsibility for feelings, thoughts, and behaviors
- Help others understand their perspective

Passive people:
- Lack self-confidence and respect
- Put others' needs ahead of their own
- Fear others' reactions (e.g., anger, rejection)
- Feel uncertain and have self-doubt

Aggressive people:
- Generate feelings of humiliation and guilt
- Disregard the rights of others
- Use "you" statements and blame others
- Lack respect for others and themselves
- Alienate others
- Speak their mind with little regard for others

Setting the Stage

Setting the right stage for assertiveness requires a nonthreatening approach consistent with verbal and nonverbal communication cues. This is particularly pivotal during stressful interactions. Stressful situations generate anxiety and distract from the issue; decrease concentration, attention, and processing of information; and impair decision-making skills. Anger and other emotions obscure what we hear and how we respond to messages, and unless they are effectively managed they can result in inappropriate behavior and even violence.

The *first step* to controlling anger and other emotions is becoming self-aware. How do you know when you are angry? It is essential to identify physical and mental reactions to anger because it is difficult to control them if they are outside your awareness zone. Physiologically anger often provokes the "fight or flight" response, which manifests as increased heart rate, respirations, blood pressure, anxiety, and muscle tension. Recognizing physiologic responses is the first step to effective anger management.

The *second step* involves taking a time out when possible to avoid escalation or aggressive or inappropriate behavior. People may question the term *time out* in an adult environment because it is normally used to help children manage disruptive behavior (e.g., temper tantrums); however, it is a very effective technique to use during high stress times when adults have temper tantrums during which they yell, throw objects, and slam doors. Time outs can be accomplished by stating "I'll be right back" or "Give me a few minutes." During time outs perform deep-breathing abdominal exercises to help control respirations (e.g., 10 slow, deep abdominal breaths), reduce heart rate and blood pressure, and facilitate "grounding." You can move yourself from a highly out of control emotional state or intense anger to a more intellectual (i.e., attentive, problem solving) state and manage intense anxiety more appropriately. (See Table 2-3 for some deep breathing exercises.)

The *third step* during this brief period is to ask, "Why am I so upset or angry? Am I overreacting?" If the anger is unjustified, calm down and refocus your energy on appropriate and constructive responses. On the other hand, if your anger is justified and the consequences are worthwhile, the *final step* is to use assertiveness to resolve the problem. Prior to talking to the individual it is important to create a nonthreatening environment. If your emotions are too intense, consider waiting until you calm down, even if it is the following day. The ability to control anger and other emotions can be learned through role playing or rehearsing desired behaviors that facilitate relaxation and modulate nonverbal cues. This can be accomplished by looking in the mirror when you are angry and noting your nonverbal cues, such

Table 2-3 Deep-Breathing Techniques

Successful deep-breathing exercises require practice and recognizing physical or emotional signs of stress, anger, or anxiety. The following steps will help you gain control over your emotions and control your emotions more effectively:

- Recognize your physiological responses to anger and stress (e.g., increased heart rate, blood pressure, and respirations; sweating; headache; dry mouth; flushing; muscle tension).
- Remove yourself from the stressful situation as appropriate.
- Find a quiet and private place.
- Pay attention to your physical reactions (noted above).
- Sit down and close your eyes.
- Focus on your breathing patterns (diaphragm and abdominal muscles):
  - Slowly inhale—Pull in your abdominal muscles while allowing your chest to rise. (Initially this pattern feels awkward, but it is actually the way we breathe when we are relaxed, such as prior to falling asleep.)
  - Exhale—Slowly breathe and allow your abdomen to move outward and your chest to slowly fall.
  - Repeat this exercise 10 times.
  - Note how when you control and decrease your respirations your entire body begins to relax, including heart rate and blood pressure. Also note the general sense of calm that comes over your body. (You are now "grounded" and in control of your emotions.)
- Once you complete the deep breaths, focus on the nature of your anger or stress.
- Is your anger legitimate or are you overreacting?
- If your anger is legitimate, return to the situation if it is important or appropriate and use assertive communication skills to address your concerns.

as an angry facial expression, sweating, frowning, or a raised brow. Once emotions and nonverbal cues are effectively managed the following are helpful steps for developing assertiveness skills:

1. Use "I or me" statements, such as "I was really upset by. . . ."
2. Describe the behaviors or concerns you have with the other person: "When you yelled at me during the morning meeting. . . ."
3. Enumerate the consequences of their behavior, including your feelings: "I felt embarrassed and angry. . . ."
4. Describe what you need or how they need to change their behavior to resolve the situation: "In the future, when you have a point to make or you disagree with me I would prefer talking about this in private or that you lower your voice and focus on issues you want me to address."

The following is an example of how a nurse can respond to an aggressive situation or person. The following numbers are used to code the conversation:

1 = I or me statement to describe behavior (empathy strengthens this statement)
2 = Describes the way you feel
3 = Consequences of the individual's behavior
4 = Describes what you need or want from the other person

Nurse: Dr. Moore, when you yell at me in front of staff I feel embarrassed and upset [#1, 2, & 3]. I understand this has been a very hectic day for the staff [#1] but in the future when you need to talk to me or ask me to do something I would appreciate you lowering your voice or not yelling, and discussing your concerns in private [#4].

During this encounter it is crucial to maintain nonthreatening body language and a safe distance (e.g., leg's length), maintain good eye contact, speak in a normal tone of voice (not whiny or abrupt), and use erect posture. Focus on the problem or behavior; avoid personal attacks or blaming or "you" statements. Sometimes people make statements such as "You upset me" or "You are responsible for this situation." "You" statements versus "I" statements, such as "I am upset at the way you treated me during the meeting" are more likely to generate a defensive response from the person you are talking to and interfere with resolving the problem. Assertiveness and effective communication are governed by the manner in which you express the message (process or nonverbal cues) and not necessarily from what you say (verbal cues). When assertive verbal content is communicated passively (through poor eye contact, whininess, or stooped posture) the message conveyed is *passiveness*. *Assertiveness* is conveyed by verbal and nonverbal congruency, or consistency between verbal (what you say) and nonverbal (body language) communication. For instance, if you express understanding that "this has been a hectic day for all of us," your voice tone, facial expression, and distance must convey genuine empathy and concerns about someone's behavior.

Regrettably, even when you are assertive there is *no guarantee* the receiver will modify his or her behavior or become more respectful. However, assertive communication engenders open and honest dialogue and provides the opportunity to problem solve and effectively resolve conflicts. Conflicts are best managed when resolved at the lowest level, meaning resolving the situation between individuals involved in the initial conflict (such as the nurse and the physician in the scenario). In the scenario, it was critical for the nurse to resolve his concerns with the physician first because they have daily contact with each other, and need to maintain trust and a healthy working relationship. In the event the behavior continues, there are several options before using the chain of command. If these options don't work, it is necessary to use the appropriate chain of command to resolve the conflict. The appropriate chain of command usually includes the line of supervision, such as talking to your immediate supervisor or nurse manager, and if the conflict is unresolved, talk to the nurse manager's supervisor and so forth.

Successful conflict resolution fosters confidence and self-respect. If you want people to respect what you say and value your ideas you must believe in or have confidence in yourself.

Remember that not all situations require a response. The decision to avoid conflict is not synonymous with passiveness when it is a conscious and well-thought-out decision based on an assessment of benefits and potential consequences.

Clarification

Clarification is necessary when the nurse needs additional information or validation of clinical data and interpretation of verbal and nonverbal communication. Appropriate questioning techniques clarify this information. Helping the client discover what he or she wants to say makes the message clearer to the nurse and client. This technique requires active and objective listening. It creates a safe and caring environment that encourages the client to express feelings and specific details concerning the present situation. The following is an example of clarification:

Client: I just lost my job and don't know what I'm going to do. As you can see my blood pressure is very high today.

Nurse: I understand losing your job is devastating. *(Displays empathy about his situation)* Tell me what lifestyle changes you've experienced since losing your job. *(Clarifies the impact of losing his job, such as financial, interpersonal)*

Client: I have a son in his first year of college and my wife blames me for not saving for his education.

Nurse: When was the last time you discussed your concerns with your wife? *(Clarifies the impact of losing job on marriage)*

Client: We seldom talk and she doesn't know how I feel about losing my job. She's in the waiting room. Do you want to talk to her?

Nurse: I am concerned about your current family stress and its effect on your blood pressure. It's a good idea to ask her to come in now so we can discuss your concerns. *(Displays empathy, imparts information, and suggests looking at his wife's perspective about the current situation)*

Client: Okay. Let me get her.

Clarifying the client's complaints about losing his job and subsequent financial and marital problems, and linking current stressors to elevated blood pressure facilitated a greater appreciation of the client's experience. Apart from feeling guilty about his son, he had problems sharing his feelings and concerns with his wife. This was an ideal time to talk to the client and his wife to also clarify her responses about the current situation.

Conflict Resolution

A **conflict** is a mental struggle arising from opposing demands or impulses. Most people associate conflicts with negativity and avoid them at all costs. They are frequently avoided and minimized due to poor communication and assertiveness skills, low self-esteem, lack of confidence, fear of losing, or feeling victimized. Conflicts are associated with the following:

- Gender issues
- Ethnicity
- Culture
- Perceptions
- Education level
- Values
- Beliefs
- Moral issues
- Self-esteem

- Stress
- Anxiety
- Language difficulties
- Socioeconomic status
- Coping style
- Ethics
- Fear
- Ageism
- Developmental stage

Conflicts can be threatening and have the propensity to incite strong and negative feelings, discord, and disagreements. In reality, they are an integral part of human interactions and relationships. Conflicts afford opportunities to exchange ideas, and to appreciate and tolerate the differences each person brings to the situation. Daily interactions with clients, coworkers, and stakeholders generate normal disagreements, disputes, and conflicts. Conflicts are frequently associated with behaviors, not people; hence we need to remain focused on the behavior, not the person's qualities and characteristics. As previously discussed, **conflict management** requires effective communication skills. A common query concerning conflicts is "If conflict resolution is so important, why do so many people walk away from conflicts?" The answer is complicated and multifaceted.

Nurses, clients, and health care providers bring a variety of human experiences, beliefs, values, and cultures to health systems. In addition, early childhood experiences with conflicts, stress, and trust along with socialization issues influence one's perception of conflict and willingness and ability to resolve it. Self-esteem, positive self-regard, confidence, and potential consequences also govern the decision to resolve or walk away from conflicts. The importance of assertiveness in resolving conflicts was previously discussed. The following dialogue demonstrates conflict resolution techniques:

Mr. Jones: When I take this medication I have sexual problems and my wife is unhappy.

Nurse: Mr. Jones I understand your concerns, but if you do not take your medication as ordered you will get sick and end up in the hospital again. *(Although adherence to medication is important, the nurse fails to empathize with the client's situation, which generates conflict.)*

Mr. Jones: I don't care. I know I need to take this medication, but I also know my body better than anyone else. I only skip doses periodically and besides, I've taken this medication long enough to know when I'm getting sick.

[The nurse insists that the client take the daily dose as prescribed, and he refuses to comply.]

Nurse: Okay Mr. Jones, I know you have been on this medication for a while and I respect your honesty in letting me know how you are taking it. Although I do not agree with the way you take your medication, I respect your honesty and understand how important it is for you to make decisions about your health. *(She recognizes the continued conflict, compromises, and negotiates with the client to address his concerns.)*

Mr. Jones: Thank you. I was concerned you would be upset and not understand how important this was to me.

Nurse: Thanks again for bringing this to my attention. Please let me know if you have more problems with your medication. I will inform your primary care provider about this and she will call you if she has further questions or concerns.

This scenario demonstrates how the nurse used assertiveness to negotiate with the client about medication adherence. Although she did not condone how he took his medication, she supported his decision to take the medication to manage symptoms and avoid relapse. She was more concerned about treatment adherence rather than stopping it because she felt he needed to take it daily as prescribed. In this scenario, the client periodically took medication to minimize sexual side effects and still managed symptoms. Although it was very important to negotiate and resolve the nurse–client conflict, it was equally important to maintain trust and openness and recognize that the decision to adhere to medication and self-manage symptoms rests with the client.

Effective conflict resolution or negotiation strengthens relationships, engenders mutual respect and trust, and fosters self-esteem, autonomy, self-efficacy, and collaboration. Predictably, poorly managed or avoided conflict reduces productivity and positive health outcomes, erodes trust and effective communication, and contributes to future conflicts.

Confrontation

Confrontation is often perceived as "beating on the table and shouting," but in reality it is a therapeutic intervention that requires control and focus on specific behaviors and aggression. Confrontation is a therapeutic technique used to point out incongruence between what is said and one's behavior. Because of misperceptions, it is often uncomfortable to the client and the inexperienced nurse. Motivational theorists and mental health professionals view confrontation as an integral part of interpersonal relationships and assert that when people recognize discrepancies they can make healthy behavioral changes (Miller, 1985; Miller & Rollnick, 1991). Because confrontation evokes intense anxiety, is uncomfortable, and carries misgivings, it is often underutilized as an important communication tool.

The following demonstrates the usefulness of confrontation between a nurse and client. The nurse has worked with Mr. Ekpong in the diabetic clinic since he was diagnosed with Type II diabetes 12 months ago. He is in for a follow-up appointment for diabetes today.

Nurse: Good morning Mr. Ekpong. I noticed your HgbA1c lab today is higher than at your last visit.

Mr. Ekpong: I don't know why because I take my medication and follow my diet as instructed. *(Defensive)*

Nurse: Well, I understand, but prior to this visit your HgbA1c had decreased and today it's pretty high. *(Confronts about abnormal HgbA1c based on previous results, which is incongruent with following diet and other treatment considerations)*

Mr. Ekpong: *(Raises voice)* It sounds like you don't believe me!

Nurse: *(Remains calm and focused)* It's not that I don't believe you, but based on your blood work you may be doing something different with your diet or medication. I am really concerned about it and your health and want to make sure you stay on the right track. *(Confronts again because of client's defensiveness, but focuses on results [behavior] without criticizing the client)*

Mr. Ekpong: I know you care what happens to me. I apologize and confess that during the holidays I ate a lot of desserts and did not exercise as often as I should have. I'm sorry I raised my voice.

Nurse: Thanks for your honesty Mr. Ekpong. It's difficult for most of us to stick to our diets during the holidays. However, it is important to know why your lab results changed to understand if your medication needs to be changed. As you know, even though it's difficult, it is important to adhere to your diet, medication, and exercise program to maintain your health. In the future, please let me know if this is a problem. *(Responded in a positive manner to reinforce honesty about diet during the holidays)*

Mr. Ekpong: Thanks for understanding. I thought you were going to be mad at me for "slipping."

Nurse: Not at all. By the way, your other lab studies look pretty good.

Confrontation is a powerful communication tool and, when used appropriately by specifically focusing on behavior and not the individual, maintains communication and minimizes defensiveness and anxiety. This example demonstrates the importance of remaining calm and focusing on the client's behavior while avoiding defensive or angry counter-reactions.

Focusing

Focusing is the process of clarifying a perception or pointing out aspects of the conversation. This process fosters attentiveness and helps the nurse gather relevant data to validate a specific point. It facilitates quality dialogue and helps the overly anxious or easily distracted client concentrate on the subject matter.

The following scenario depicts focusing. Mary is a 21-year-old student recently diagnosed with Crohn's disease who is in for a medication review follow-up.

Nurse: Mary you look pretty down today. What's going on? *(The nurse attempts to focus on and assess the meaning of client's behaviors and demeanor)*

Mary: Nothing.

Nurse: You look sadder today than during your last visit and I noticed your eyes are red and puffy. *(By focusing and using explicit physical details to explain her concerns she conveys astute observational skills and empathy.)*

Mary: I just had a bad night!

Nurse: A bad night? Tell me how long you've had problems sleeping. *(Focusing encourages the client to provide more details about sleeping patterns and define "bad night.")*

Mary: Oh, the past few weeks. I go to bed okay, but wake up about 2 AM and can't go back to sleep.

Nurse: What other changes have you had over the past few weeks? *(Focusing helps the nurse clarify and assess the client's present situation.)*

Mary: My boyfriend broke up with me because of my medical problem.

Nurse: What do you mean medical problem? *(Focusing again helps the nurse clarify and assess the client's situation.)*

Mary: I told him about the possible surgery and he just couldn't take it.

Nurse: Please tell me more about the way you've been feeling since the breakup.

Although the client's visit was about her medical problems, she was very stressed and upset or even depressed about the recent relationship breakup. Obviously, the nurse suspected Mary was pretty distraught, and by focusing on her complaints was able to validate her concerns by gathering specific information concerning underlying psychosocial stressors and possible treatment considerations. It is essential for the nurse to *be with the client* and providing venues, such as focusing, to explore and understand his or her experiences related to illness.

Giving or Imparting Information

Giving or **imparting information** is an integral part of nursing. This process involves giving facts when the client asks for or seeks information. Through health education, informed consent, orientation, and other methods, the nurse can devise individualized interventions that allay fears and anxiety and promote treatment adherence.

Mr. Schultz is an older adult who was been recently diagnosed with Parkinson's disease. He is anxious and concerned that he will be unable to walk due to physical symptoms of his illness. The nurse has opportunities to mitigate his anxiety and concerns through emotional support, empathy, and health education.

Nurse: Mr. Schultz, I see you have been started on a new medication for Parkinson's disease.

Mr. Schultz: I understand about Parkinson's disease, but I need more information about my medication.

Nurse: What is your understanding about your medication, including how it works?

Mr. Schultz: Isn't the medication supposed to stop these tremors and stiffness?

Nurse: Yes, it is. I'll review each medication again and explain any side effects or symptoms to report.

Mr. Schultz: I am so glad because I want to get better.

This dialogue demonstrates the significance of client-centered health education (imparting information). Imparting information ensures shared decision making, reduces anxiety, and facilitates informed consent. It engenders trust and mutual respect, which are key issues in treatment adherence and clinical health outcomes.

Humor

Humor refers to being amusing, funny, or comical to express feelings and thoughts in a manner comfortable to oneself and others. Nurses may be surprised by the frequency with which some clients use humor to poke fun at themselves. It is helpful to note that humor often alleviates stress and anxiety and helps express very challenging thoughts and feelings. Appropriate use of humor enriches interpersonal relationships, reduces stress, minimizes cultural differences, and helps communicate difficult messages.

Humor is underused as a therapeutic communication tool. The chief health benefits of humor have been historically acknowledged, but only anecdotally because quantifying its effectiveness has been difficult. However, even though results are tentative, there is growing evidence of the therapeutic qualities of humor and laughter (Martin, 2001). Researchers state that humor and laughter may be effective self-care strategies to cope with stress and provide physical relief of muscle tension (Wooten, 1996), to improve natural killer (NK) cell activity (Bennett, Zeller, Rosenberg, & McCann, 2003), and thereby to improve immune function (MacDonald, 2004).

Laughter stimulates physiologic processes. It strengthens heart rate and respirations, reduces stress hormones, and activates endorphins, the body's own natural morphine-like chemicals, which improve mood (Hassed, 2001). Collectively, laughter and humor are stress busters with healing properties. When used appropriately, humor provides a temporary distraction from stressful or overwhelming feelings and fears. Appropriate use of humor requires acceptance by the client, which is conveyed through verbal and nonverbal communication. The use of humor should be avoided if it is offensive or culturally insensitive, or during a catastrophic or grave situation. Although humor has stress-reducing and healing properties, when used inappropriately it can be destructive, such as when a client pokes fun at her- or himself as a "put down" to galvanize low self-esteem. Nurses must discourage the destructive use of humor and encourage clients to focus on strengths and positive attributes. Naturally, more rigorous and theoretically sound research is necessary before conclusive statements can be made regarding the health benefits of laughter and humor.

Negotiation

Negotiation is an integral part of working with people. People are often unaware of how often they negotiate. For instance, you would never pay the stated dealer's price for an automobile. Certainly the car dealer expects you to ask for the best deal. Cars often have a higher markup simply because negotiation is expected. This also occurs in health care systems when purchasers and contractors negotiate for the best price. More and more nurses find themselves in positions that require negotiation skills to handle complex client needs, ensure appropriate and client-centered health care, and provide equitable resource allocation.

Furthermore, technological advances and the explosion of information systems have created a very competitive health care arena. Dwindling resources and high-stress work environments also contribute to interpersonal conflict and tension. Negotiation with the client fosters shared or participatory decision making and acknowledges his or her autonomy. Negotiation is critical and requires *give and take* communication processes to diffuse tension and effectively resolve conflicts and stressful interpersonal interactions. As brokers of health care, nurses must use negotiation skills to navigate health care across the continuum. The nurse must be able to work effectively with others. Negotiation requires team-building communication skills and knowledge of group or team dynamics to balance the needs of clients, families, or caregivers with available resources and expertise as a team member. (An extensive discussion of negotiation is included in Chapter 5, Professional Development: Leading Through Effective Communication.)

How can you become a good negotiator? You may already have negotiating skills, but how often are you using them? Unless you are confident and assertive and have good listening skills, you will have difficulty negotiating. Although negotiation occurs daily, it is not an easy process. As previously mentioned, interpersonal skills are the basis of successful negotiation. Key questions to answer before you decide to negotiate are:

- What is the chief issue to resolve, and how important is it?
- Do I have an understanding of the full picture? (In other words, what additional information do I need from others?)
- What is my relationship with key players or partners?
- What do I hope to gain or accomplish?
- What resources do I need to successfully negotiate or resolve key issues?
- How much am I willing to invest in the process?

Active listening is especially important during stressful interactions because it helps the nurse negotiate more effectively by hearing others' perspectives. It guides attentive listening regarding what we hear and what others say. Often, poor listening skills or inattentiveness along with interruptions result in conflict and necessitate negotiation. Paying close attention to what is said and periodically clarifying, restating, and paraphrasing demonstrate respect and foster trust. Moreover, it embraces others' concerns, needs, and perceptions and builds healthy interpersonal relationships. Successful negotiation also requires a trusting environment, sound nurse–client communication, and assertiveness that facilitates the social interaction crucial to resolving problems or other conflicts (Yamashita, Forchuk, & Mound, 2005). An example of this concept is working with a client with hypertension to enhance medication adherence. Initially, the nurse must establish rapport and trust, listen to and understand the client's concerns, provide health education to the client and family, and negotiate ways to ensure safe and high-quality clinical outcomes. Clients often give numerous reasons for nonadherence to treatment; before making assumptions, it is important to understand the client's experience, health practices, and motivation to adhere to treatment. This provides a position of power for negotiating and using shared decision making with the client to discuss health care needs, mutually established goals, and holistic treatment planning. (See Research Study 2-1 on page 94.)

Overall, effective negotiation is a win-win process that facilitates shared decision making, problem solving, and conflict resolution through a give-and-take approach. In successful negotiation, all parties must feel their issues and positions are understood. The following criteria provide further guidance in negotiation:

- Uses a practical decision-making process
- Is cost-effective, client-centered, and evidence-based
- Improves or sustains healthy communication and interpersonal relationships

Questioning

Questioning is an essential communication tool. It builds rapport and trust, encourages shared decision making, elicits important health data, and helps the nurse understand the client's experience, preferences, and needs. In addition, seeking feedback and securing information validates or tests assumptions concerning verbal and nonverbal communication. Some clients are hesitant to speak or to divulge information, especially during an initial encounter, unless privacy is ensured. It is important for the nurse to provide a quiet, private, and safe environment without unnecessary interruptions. Due to normal anxiety during an initial encounter, it is equally important to begin the assessment with a statement such as "I noticed you seem to be nervous about talking to me, and I wonder what I can do to make you more comfortable?" The nurse is challenged to maintain a balance, letting the client provide reasons for seeking treatment and prompting through questions that yield important clinical data. Broad open-ended questioning is suggested initially, leading to more direct and detailed questioning at the end of the assessment.

Open-ended questions are more likely to provide quality feedback because they elicit answers to "what," "when," "how," and "where" concerning the client's behavior. In comparison, closed-ended queries or those that yield "yes" or "no" or limited answers reduce quality responses and should be avoided or used sparingly. They are used to collect specific information such as "Are you married?", "Are you currently employed?", or "Are you safe in your home?" Avoid direct or probing questions that begin with "why" because they tend to elicit defensiveness and argumentativeness, as well as noncommittal responses. The following are examples of open-ended and closed-ended questioning.

Open-Ended Questioning

Nurse: Good evening, Mr. Effiong. My name is Sherry and I am your nurse today. What's brought you in today?

Client: I'm having chest pains and my doctor asked me to come to the emergency room.

Nurse: How long have you had chest pains?

Client: They started yesterday, but I thought it was just indigestion.

Nurse: Mr. Effiong, please describe your chest pain.

Client: They are sharp and hit me in the center of my chest. They are worse after meals, but they come and go.

Nurse: Are you having chest pain right now?

Client: No, I don't have any right now.

Nurse: When you are in pain, please describe it on a scale of 1–10 [1 = minimal, 10 = severe].

Client: It's about 6–7.

Nurse: How long does each episode last?

Client: About 2–3 minutes.

Nurse: What about your breathing?

Client: Even though I get short winded when I have chest pain, my breathing is fine now.

Nurse: What kind of medications have you taken today?

Client: My doctor told me to take aspirin. I took it about 30 minutes ago. Nurse, am I going to die?

Nurse: Mr. Effiong, I understand your fears of dying and they are normal under the present circumstances. You made the right decision to come to the emergency room today. We are going to do everything to evaluate and treat your chest pain. Your doctor will see you soon.

Client: Thank you. I am so nervous, but I know you all are going to take care of me.

In this scenario, the nurse was able to elicit specific and detailed information about the client's condition by asking open-ended questions, which yielded an important and detailed description of chest pain, breathing patterns, and medications. Not all clients give specific information when asked open-ended questions. This supportive and caring environment also helped the client express fears and be reassured that he was in the right place.

Closed-Ended Questioning

Although closed-ended questions should be used sparingly, they can elicit specific information, such as demographics, presence and absence of specific symptoms, or thoughts. The chief limitations of closed-ended questions include:

- They are guided by the nurse.
- They restrict the client's ability to freely answer questions or express feelings.
- The focus is narrowed to "yes" or "no" or limited responses.

Note the limited range of questions and answers and diminished opportunities to respond in the following discussion:

Nurse: Mr. Jones, are you having chest pains?

Client: Yes.

Nurse: Did your doctor instruct you to come to the emergency room?

Client: Yes.

Nurse: Did you take any medications today?

Client: Yes.

When used exclusively, closed-ended questions yield minimal information concerning the quality of the client's symptoms, thoughts, and behavior. As a general rule, closed-ended and open-ended questions must be balanced and used appropriately to clearly comprehend the client's perceptions and symptoms, and allow full expression of his or her experience. The following are examples of appropriate closed-ended questions:

- How many children do you have?
- Do you use a helmet when driving your motorcycle?
- Do you smoke cigarettes?
- Did you take your medication this morning?
- Are you safe in your home?
- Have you ever been arrested?
- Have you ever tried to harm yourself or other?

When closed-ended questions are the sole queries they only provide part of the necessary information needed to complete the nursing assessment.

However, when followed by open-ended questions they yield invaluable clinical information. Balancing closed-ended questions with open-ended questions enables the nurse to clarify and gather more data concerning the client's health status.

Reflection

Reflection or reflective listening is one of the most difficult communication skills. It requires astute active listening skills and awareness of nonverbal responses. Apart from active listening, it requires responsiveness to or reasonable guesses of what the client means. Assumptions are guesses that must be validated by the client. Reflection uses statements based on client comments to confirm assertions or assumptions, as noted in the following encounter.

During a patient's initial visit in a primary care dermatology clinic, the nurse gathers information about recent stressors. The client states he has had marital problems for the past 3–6 months. He also admits his wife complains he spends too much time on the Internet and not enough time with her. Even though your hunch links the client's dermatologic problems to marital discord, it is important to avoid drawing premature conclusions and validating your assumptions, as noted in the following conversation:

Client: I spend too much time on the Internet and not enough with my wife.

Nurse: You feel you are spending too much time on the Internet. *(Statement, not an assumption)*

Client: Yes. My wife complains every evening because I am on the computer.

Nurse: She is angry because you spend too much time on the Internet. *(Restatement or reflective listening)*

Client: You bet! She slams doors and refuses to cook sometimes.

Nurse: And you are concerned about your marriage. *(A guess at his feelings [reflecting feelings or an "interpretation"])*

Client: Yes.

Reflection or reflective listening enabled the nurse to elicit important information from the client by simply making statements about what he thought the client meant. It was less threatening than probing questions, yet yielded important information about the client's marital situation.

Self-Disclosure

The precise role of **self-disclosure** in the nurse–client relationship is unclear. However, Jourard's (1964) theory suggests that an optimal level of self-disclosure is essential for healthy relationships, and is governed by the nature of the relationship with others. The client's needs, rather than the nurse's, govern self-disclosure. For instance, personal information, such as current medications, medical problems, and age, may be shared with selected close friends and family; less personal information such as name, discipline, or educational background may be shared with others as appropriate. It is vital to note that there are situations in which self-disclosure is inappropriate. The nurse should *never* use self-disclosure to resolve personal problems or as a basis for personal gratification. The decision to disclose information to the client must be carefully considered, and used only to advance the client's health goals based on the needs of the client (rather than the nurse), appropriateness, and timeliness. Before self-disclosing it is very important to assess your motivation and its impact on the client. The following situation is an example in which the nurse may choose to self-disclose to improve an interpersonal relationship and model adaptive behaviors.

A mother comes to the pediatric clinic and expresses concerns about her ill child; during the course of her visit the following dialogue between and the nurse and mother occurs.

Mother: Are you a mother? Do you really understand what I'm going through?

Nurses: Yes, I am a mother and you have a right to be concerned about your child. I understand how difficult this must be for you.

In this situation, the nurse must remain calm and reassure the parent that everything is being done to care for her child. Overall, appropriate self-disclosure is an important nursing intervention and communication skill that ensures and maintains healthy boundaries between the nurse and the client. It fosters trust, conveys empathy, encourages shared decision making and motivation, reduces fears, and normalizes the client's experiences (Enns, 1997; Antai-Otong, 2006; Fay, 2002). However, when used inappropriately, self-disclosure is the most dangerous communication technique for blurring boundaries and must be used cautiously. Inappropriate self-disclosure includes sharing personal information, such as home address, telephone number, or email address.

Silence

Many people feel uncomfortable with **silence**. However, when used appropriately it is an important therapeutic intervention that helps the client to collect and organize thoughts and respond to queries or aspects of the conversation. Sometimes silence indicates distrust or hostility, and it is imperative to avoid "pushing" the client to respond or talk in light of the unpredictable nature of her or his underlying thought processes. Other times the client values silence as part of his or her culture. Some clients prefer less talk and are comfortable with silence. Pressing clients to talk or respond is disrespectful, conveys impatience, and increases the risk of hostility, distrust, and verbal and physical violence. Other times silence means the client has lost his or her train of thought and has actually forgotten the query. Under these circumstances the nurse must be patient, calm, and supportive. It may also be necessary to repeat the question or aspects of the conversation to re-engage the client after silence. Silence may also be uncomfortable to the nurse who feels it is important to maintain dialogue. Normally silence lasts only a few minutes, but it may feel like hours.

During silence, focus on how you respond to silence—are you nervous, do you experience shortness of breath or sweaty palms, or are you fearful you may say the wrong thing or upset the client? Or do you feel comfortable, as evidenced by a calm demeanor and physical responses. If you experience anxiety or tension, take several deep breaths (slowly inhale and exhale) and allow yourself to relax and focus on the situation.

Equally significant is determining the usefulness of silence to the client and when to interrupt the silence. It is difficult to determine the best time to use silence, but understanding its benefits and limitations can guide the nurse in using this communication technique. Appropriate use of silence promotes calmness and accessibility to the client who may be struggling to organize thoughts and responses to difficult emotions and situations. More importantly, this brief role-playing exercise promotes self-awareness and understanding of personal reactions to silence and how to manage uncomfortable situations. Limitations associated with extended silence include inefficient use of time, avoidance of important patient disclosure, and increased anxiety in the nurse and client.

Summarizing

Summarizing involves focusing on salient points of the nurse-client interaction. It enables the nurse and client to list major points of an encounter, such as recommendations or suggestions, clarifies disagreements, and allows time to reflect on feelings, thoughts, or discussions. It reflects active listening skills, conveys caring and acceptance, and fosters a therapeutic nurse–client relationship. It enables the nurse to validate clinical findings and understand the client's problems, goals, and experiences.

Nurse: Ms. Garcia, it looks like this has been a pretty difficult year for you.

Ms. Garcia: Yes, it has. As I mentioned, I was diagnosed with diabetes several months ago and just found out I have to take insulin shots.

Nurse: Your concerns about your health and learning how to give yourself insulin injections are certainly understandable.

Ms. Garcia: That is good to hear because I never liked needles and I am very anxious about giving myself insulin.

Nurse: Let's review the steps of giving your injection again. I know how anxious you are, but believe it or not with time this gets easier.

Ms. Garcia: Yes, I am anxious, but I believe I can do this.

The nurse and client summarized the salient issues of this interaction involving newly diagnosed diabetes and fear of injections. The client was able to validate normal reactions to this situation and feel empowered through health education to manage a chronic disease. It also helped the nurse validate the client's understanding and meaning of her illness, feelings, motivation, and treatment considerations. More importantly, the nurse used this holistic approach to actively engage the client in verbalizing her thoughts and fears, reducing anxiety, and integrating health education into self-management skills.

Verbalizing the Implied

Verbalizing the implied involves clarifying what the person implied or insinuated in order to understand the message or conversation. For example, a follow-up visit with a client with hypertension shows elevated blood pressure, and she looks anxious and stressed. Implied behaviors include nonverbal and verbal cues that communicate what the client fails to explicate. Based on an assumption concerning the meaning of these behaviors, the nurse states what she believes is the real message. The following demonstrates this technique:

Nurse: Mrs. Marshall, your blood pressure is higher this time. What changes have you experienced since your last visit?

Mrs. Marshall: My 36-year-old son moved in several months ago after losing his job. I don't know how long he plans to live with us.

Nurse: You sound pretty stressed about your present living situation.

Mrs. Marshall: What makes you say that?

Nurse: Well your blood pressure is higher this time and it sounds like your present living situation is pretty stressful. How can I assist you?

Mrs. Marshall: Just listening helps. I feel guilty about complaining.

Nurse: Obviously this is a stressful time. Tell me more.

Active listening and attentiveness provided an opening for communication that validated a relationship among the client's elevated blood pressure, stress, and current living conditions. The nurse's willingness to listen, display concern, and ask relevant questions created a warm, supportive, and accepting environment conducive to sharing and expressing feelings. Furthermore, through active listening and attentiveness the nurse verbalized and clarified the meaning of the client's elevated blood pressure and obvious anxiety and stress.

Verbalizing the implied validates the nurse's perception and understanding of the client's message, conveys empathy, and strengthens the nurse–client relationship.

Therapeutic communication techniques are critical to successful nurse–client relationships. They enable the nurse to approach each situation assertively with respect to her- or himself and others. Prepared with self-assuredness and confidence the nurse can actively listen, clarify ambiguities, verbalize the implied, confront inconsistencies, and collaborate with the client, family or caregiver, and staff to ensure safe and high-quality health care.

This section has focused primarily on adults. Because each developmental stage has its own challenges and unique aspects, the following section centers on therapeutic communication techniques across the life span. Major areas include infancy and childhood, adolescence, families, and older adulthood.

LIFE SPAN CONSIDERATIONS

Developmental factors influence how we communicate and form relationships with others. As discussed in Chapter 1, early interactions are the basis of trust and influence the quality of long-term relationships. Cultural and psychosocial factors also influence communication patterns and trust in others. This section focuses on life span issues and the use of various therapeutic techniques to engender trust, establish rapport, impart information, and collaborate with families from infancy to older adulthood.

Infancy and Childhood

The word *infancy* stems from the Latin word for *without language*. Although infants are helpless and unable to communicate with words or language, they do communicate in other ways. The early cry during infancy permits the newborn to communicate biological needs, such as hunger, pain, frustration, or distress. Early contact through touch, tone of voice, feeding, eye contact, holding, and talking provides a venue for communication between parents or early caregivers and the infant. Early in their life, infants learn how to distinguish their parents' voices from others and communicate this through cooing to parents or crying with strangers.

Nurses caring for sick infants can also detect the infant's responses through various signs such as increased heart rate and respirations. Holding, feeding, and talking in a calm voice influence the newborn's reaction to the nurse and early caregivers, as evidenced by reduced heart rate and respirations. The ill infant may also mimic smiling or other pleasant facial expressions. Working with infants and children requires establishing therapeutic relationships with parents and caregivers; therapeutic techniques such as empathy, rapport, and active listening skills are crucial to establishing these relationships.

Toddlers gain confidence and a sense of separateness from others or autonomy by using words such as "that's mine," "me," or "you." Each subsequent stage is influenced by successful mastery of previous stages that further advance trust, autonomy, initiative, industry, and ability to form healthy interpersonal relationships with others (Erikson, 1968). A failure to master these developmental milestones contributes to mistrust, difficulty forming healthy interpersonal relationships, and problems communicating personal needs.

Like adults, children communicate verbally and nonverbally. Communication provides a venue through which to learn and maintain social interactions; gain attention; sort information about the world; reduce anxiety, alienation, and fear; and receive validation from parents and other social contacts. Moreover, because children have immature cognitive and language development, communication extends to other venues such as art, music, and play. For instance, the nurse working with an 8-year-old newly diagnosed with juvenile diabetes is challenged to establish rapport with the child and parents while recognizing the impact of anxiety and fears that may detract from their learning processes.

Therapeutic techniques such as those already mentioned are vital to helping the youth and family cope with and understand illness and treatment options. Nurses can also strengthen interactions with children and their families by using the following techniques:

- Maintain eye contact.
- Approach the child in a gentle and calm manner.
- Use play therapy, storytelling, painting, and other strategies to understand the child's experience.
- Encourage expression of feelings and fears.
- Listen attentively.
- Use words understandable to the child and parents.
- Use age-appropriate dialogue.
- Avoid defensiveness with parents.
- Validate assumptions about nonverbal communication.

Family Issues

Children are part of a larger family system and community. Concurrent communication with parents is crucial. The child–parent relationship and communication patterns influence acceptance of the child's illness and ability to cope and receive support. Quality communication with children also requires establishing and maintaining rapport and communication with families. Each family has its own communication patterns, parenting skills, culture and ethnicity, individual choices, and beliefs about health practices. Dynamic communication patterns challenge nurses to embrace the influence of a variety of factors on relationships with children, youth, and families and use therapeutic techniques to establish rapport, engender trust, and understand the meaning of their experiences.

Typically, parents are extremely stressed and experience a wide range of emotions when their child is ill or hospitalized. Normal stress reactions include guilt, anxiety, anger, fear, sadness, and overwhelming helplessness, which often manifest as uncooperativeness, blaming, and argumentativeness. These are very difficult times for both the child and parents, and it is crucial to avoid personalizing stress reactions. It is important to display empathy and understanding and to set limits when appropriate (e.g., discourage verbal abuse). The following is an example of an interpersonal conflict with a parent.

Jeremy, a 10-year-old boy, has been hospitalized for a diagnostic workup to rule out a serious heart condition. His parents are very upset about the preliminary findings and diagnosis and begin yelling at the nurse and blaming the hospital for not bringing the child's meal on time.

Parent: I hate this hospital. No one seems to care about my son's meal being served on time!

Nurse: I understand you are upset about the results of your child's test, but it is very difficult for me to help or listen when you yell. Jeremy just returned to the room and I have already ordered his tray.

Parent: You really don't care about my child. Just bring the tray when it comes.

Nurse: I know how scary this situation must be, let's talk some more after his meal.

Parent: You really don't know how I feel!

Nurse: You're right, I don't, but I can imagine how difficult the past few days have been for you, your husband, and Jeremy. I can arrange to talk to both of you this evening if you like.

Parent: I don't think it'll help, but I'm willing to try.

Obviously the parent is upset and angry, but has problems recognizing that her feelings are normal, although she expresses them inappropriately. Through rapport, empathy, reflection, and assertiveness, the nurse conveyed empathy, remained calm, and expressed understanding of the parent's concerns. She did not personalize the attacks, yet she set verbal limits by maintaining her composure and redirecting the parent's anger. Helping parents and families cope with difficult situations is governed by trust, respect, and the nurse–client relationship. Healthy interpersonal relationships with the child and family can reduce stress, normalize reactions, and impart information and education that strengthen the family's coping skills.

Adolescence

Adolescence is a turbulent period—more so than any other developmental stage. It marks the transition from childhood to adulthood. The adolescent not only faces enormous biological changes, but also must confront psychosocial issues and determine his or her sense of identity. Peer pressure and the need to identify with others are particularly significant during this period. The ability to master these challenges, use effective communication skills, and form interpersonal relationships are determined by early interactions with parents or caregivers. Early relationships govern the ability to form and maintain high-quality and meaningful relationships, a sense of identity, and close intimate adult relationships. The quality of the marital or couple dyad (parents) and their parenting skills impact the family's ability to cope and manage stress.

Apart from these normal developmental stressors, the adolescent experiences struggles and turmoil between self and parents to transition to adulthood. Family conflicts generally stem from disagreements about chores, blasting music, dress or style, and curfews, which are normal aspects of adolescence. Parents and teens negotiate some of these issues while maintaining the integrity of the family unit. The family's ability to manage and cope with these stressors centers on the youth's mastery of previous developmental tasks, particularly trust.

Additional social issues confronting adolescents and their families include teenage pregnancy, socioeconomic challenges, and divorce. Family support is critical for all age groups, but is particularly essential for the successful outcome of diverse social issues during adolescence. The transition from parenthood to grandparenthood is frequently unexpected and complicated for low-income and single parents. It is necessary for the nurse to identify the various stressors for both parents and the adolescent and design client- and family-centered interventions that support complex family dynamics (Dallas, 2004).

Although self-esteem and self-concept are normal developmental issues during adolescence, communication difficulties associated with transitions from adolescence to adulthood also confront the youth. Knowledge of normal developmental issues and potential struggles confronting adolescents opens up lines of communication.

Difficulty establishing trust with the nurse due to fear that information will be shared with parents may jeopardize communication with adolescents. Many are concerned about confidentiality and are hesitant to share personal information. Trust must be established along with honesty about confidentiality. Issues such as harm to self and others must be shared with parents and appropriate staff to ensure safety.

Illnesses during adolescence also place tremendous burden on the adolescent and family. Working with an adolescent's physical and mental health problems challenges the nurse to integrate life span or developmental concepts into a plan of care that establishes trust, ensures safety, and educates the youth and family about illness. Involving the youth in youth groups that address health care issues provides additional support and opportunities to communicate feelings, fears, and concerns. As mentioned earlier, the bases of nurse–client interactions include trust, respect, acceptance, empathy, and shared decision making with the youth and family.

Middle Adulthood

This period finds adults at the peak of their careers and concerned with guiding and influencing the next generation (Erikson, 1968). For many adults this is the most productive time of their life, offering opportunities to fulfill lifelong aspirations and influence the family's next generation. Major challenges during this period range from raising young children, coping with adolescents, handling adolescents or children leaving home or going to a university, facing age-related changes, coming to terms with grandparenthood, and caring for aging parents and adult children. Responsibilities and stress escalate during middle adulthood, as does vulnerability to serious medical and mental health problems.

As middle-aged adults enter the health care arena, the nurse must identify issues unique to this developmental stage. Important communication skills are similar to other developmental stages and include establishing trust and rapport, using active listening, and imparting information. Of particular importance to individuals in this developmental stage is control over one's life and health. Nurses can advance personal control, self-efficacy, and self-management through collaborative relationships and shared decision making to devise individualized care. Like previous developmental stages, this period is governed by the quality of interactions with early caregivers and parents. It also determines how middle-aged adults cope with older adulthood.

Older Adulthood

People are living longer and face diverse challenges associated with aging. The primary developmental task during older adulthood is integrity versus despair (Erikson, 1968). This stage is a culmination of previous life span tasks that influence the meaning of life and contributions to society. Developmental challenges are also impacted by normal age-related changes, significant losses, and major medical problems. The quality of lifelong relationships, level of self-esteem, culture and ethnicity, physical and mental health status, and quality of support systems impact nurse–client relationships with older adults. In addition to assessing age-specific issues of older adulthood, it is vital to determine the role and quality of families, caregivers, and significant others.

Today's societies place tremendous emphasis on youth and devalue the uniqueness of aging. In societies and families where older adults are revered and valued, emphasis is placed on their knowledge, wisdom, and role in the family. Apart from ageism, older adults must adapt to age-related biological changes. Nurses must identify variables that jeopardize individualized health care, reduce stereotyping, and implement strategies to ensure dignity, acceptance, and respect; avoid ageism; and embrace life experiences and contributions to society and wisdom.

Interpersonal relationships and therapeutic communication techniques in older adulthood are similar to other developmental stages. Age-related changes such as vision and hearing deficits can be minimized by speaking slowly, being more patient, allowing time to respond, and directly facing the client to ensure eye contact and understanding. Cultural factors and ethnicity play key roles in how older adults communicate problems and express feelings. Storytelling or reminiscence is an important family ritual and socialization in some cultures. Through storytelling, the family's legacy and uniqueness are communicated to the next generation. This unique style of communication also helps the nurse gain insight into the heritage, perspectives, and life experiences of diverse cultures (Bailey & Tilley, 2002; de Vries, Suedfeld, Krell, Blando, & Southard, 2005; Shellman, 2004). It helps clients from various cultures to cope with serious illness. Encouraging storytelling conveys respect and appreciation of the older adult's life experiences, health practices, and contributions to society. Embracing the distinctiveness of older adults is crucial to helping them maintain their spirituality and hope through therapeutic and healing communication.

CRITICAL THINKING QUESTION

Mr. Martinelli is an 80-year-old widower recently admitted to the Geriatric Extended Care Unit after a hip replacement. During morning rounds he yells, "I want to take my bath in the evening. Yesterday I was told I had to bathe in the morning. No one listens to me and I'm tired of it!"

Question: What is the most appropriate response to Mr. Martinelli?

  a. Mr. Martinelli, I understand how difficult it is to be in the hospital. I will arrange for you to have your bath in the evening. What else can I do to make your stay more comfortable?

  b. Mr. Martinelli, please lower your voice. It is very difficult for me to help when you shout. Now, what else do you need this morning?

  c. Mr. Martinelli, we have limited staff on the evening shift and you must take your bath as scheduled. Can I assist you with anything else?

  d. Mr. Martinelli, please lower your voice because we have sick people on this floor. I will talk to the evening nurse to see if we can arrange for you to bathe on that shift.

Answer: The correct answer is a. It recognizes age-related changes in an 80-year-old related to possible hearing loss. Unless the yelling is accompanied by other aggressive nonverbal cues, the client yelling may not be indicative of aggression. The response reflects the difficulty some older clients have saying they are afraid or fearful. It also reflects respect for the client's individual need to take his bath in the evening. This approach obviates anxiety and ensures dignity and integrity.

The other responses are incorrect or inappropriate. Although b and d address the issue of yelling, they offer little empathy about the client's request to bathe in the evening. Answer c reflects a lack of sensitivity and empathy.

CHAPTER SUMMARY

Therapeutic communication is central to nursing care. It is the foundation of all nurse–client interactions and creates opportunities to establish trust, gather relevant client data, collaborate with clients and staff, and formulate diagnoses and client-centered interventions. Therapeutic communication techniques, such as active listening, acceptance, assertiveness, conflict resolution, and negotiation, are essential components of nurse–client relationships. This is particularly important in a changing society; the transformation of health care systems and advances in telecommunications have drastically changed how people communicate. Nurses are in pivotal positions and must create innovative communication approaches, such as using video telephone conferences, the Internet, email, telehealth, and messaging devices, in client homes to create nurse–client relationships across the life span and within diverse cultures.

Effective communication techniques extend beyond the nurse–client relationship and include safe and productive work relationships. Assertive communication provides the foundation of healthy work relationships. It ensures open and honest communication that facilitates respect for self and others and effective conflict resolution and positive clinical outcomes.

The ability to establish relationships and communicate with others is governed by life span issues that impact self-confidence, trust, and reliance on others. Life span issues are an integral part of all communication. Nurses are poised to interact with individuals across the life span, ranging from children and their parents to older adults. It is imperative to understand the use of therapeutic techniques, such as active listening and empathy to create supportive and quality relationships and understand the client's experiences regardless of age.

SUGGESTIONS FOR CLINICAL AND EXPERIENTIAL ACTIVITIES

1. Invite a communications expert to do a series of lectures on assertiveness training, negotiation, and conflict resolution. Training should involve didactic discussions, role-playing, and rehearsals.
2. Use case histories of difficult client situations as a learning tool to address communication issues and communication techniques.
3. Prepare a scenario regarding a difficult or uncomfortable situation and identify various therapeutic techniques to resolve the situation.
4. Explore opportunities for self-awareness, such as what is appropriate to share with a client, how to respond to a client who asks for a date, or how to work with an individual from a different culture or ethnicity. Identify personal reactions to these situations and ways to manage them.
5. Role-play each therapeutic technique and ask other students or participants to critique it.

END-OF-CHAPTER QUESTIONS

1. You are the new nurse on an inpatient medical-surgical unit. During morning report one of your coworkers raises her voice and accuses you of leaving an unsigned progress note. What is the most appropriate response?
    a. I'm sorry. I am pretty new and appreciate you bringing this to my attention.
    b. Mary, let's talk about this after report.
    c. I don't appreciate you embarrassing me like this.
    d. Remain silent because you are the new person on the unit.
2. Which of the following behaviors is characteristic of active listening?
    a. Leaning forward and limiting eye contact
    b. Paraphrasing or restating
    c. Making corrections when obvious misunderstanding occurs
    d. Focusing on verbal communication
3. Mr. Rodriquez is a 45-year-old married man seen in primary care with a diagnosis of rheumatoid arthritis. He complains of difficulty sleeping because of chronic pain. Which of the following statements is a barrier to active listening?
    a. Why did you wait so long to seek treatment?
    b. I'm sorry, I need to get this call.
    c. Tell me about your living situation.
    d. All of the above.
4. Assertive communication is an important therapeutic communication technique. Which of the following statements best describes assertiveness?
    a. I am upset because this is the second time you've been late this week.
    b. You make me angry every time you ask that question.
    c. What can I do to keep you from being so upset?
    d. None of the above.
5. Open-ended questions are more likely to elicit quality feedback than closed-ended questions. Which of the following questions is open-ended?
    a. How old are you?
    b. Are you married?
    c. What brought you in today?
    d. Is this your first visit to primary care?
6. Reflective listening is one of the most difficult communication skills. During a recent visit with Mr. Jones he expresses concerns about his blood pressure. Which of the following shows reflective listening?

    a. Sounds like you need to change you blood pressure medication.
    b. You are worried about your blood pressure.
    c. I understand how you must feel.
    d. You have a right to be concerned about your blood pressure.

7. Mary is a 21-year-old mother of two who is being seen at a community-based clinic for an evaluation of abdominal pain. While asking questions about her symptoms she becomes silent. What is the most appropriate response to a client who is silent?
    a. Rephrase and ask the question again.
    b. Allow her time to organize her thoughts.
    c. Excuse yourself for a few minutes.
    d. Let her know you have other clients waiting.

8. Appropriate self-disclosure is an important communication technique. Which of the following is inappropriate self-disclosure?
    a. Acknowledging your marital status
    b. Giving your telephone number to a client
    c. Having your diploma or other academic achievements in view
    d. Refusing to give your spouse's name to a client

9. Jennifer is a 16-year-old seen in the school health clinic for flu-like symptoms. While obtaining her health history she admits her parents are unaware that she uses birth control pills. Which of the following is an important part of establishing a therapeutic relationship with this client?
    a. Maintaining confidentiality about non-life-threatening issues
    b. Letting her know she needs to talk to her parents about birth control pills
    c. Asking if she is sexually active
    d. Promising that everything she shares with you is confidential

Answers

9. a
8. b
7. b
6. b
5. c
4. a
3. d
2. b
1. b

Research Study 2–1

Title: Negotiating Dyadic Identity between Caregivers and Care Receivers Coeling. H. V., Biordi, D. L., & Theis, S. L. (2003). *Image. Journal of Nursing Scholarship,* 35, 21–25.

Purpose: To describe the ways in which caregivers and their care receivers in a nursing home negotiate dyadic parameters that impacted how they adapted the care experience in their lives, and to suggest theory based on the data.

Method: Caregivers and care receivers were interviewed simultaneously and separately by researchers concerning their care experiences. Data from these interviews were used to determine how their experiences were adapted into their everyday life. A qualitative analysis of these responses defined dyadic identity (a mutually agreed upon caregiving relationship determined by a set of rules involving negotiation that facilitated informal care of a loved one who used nursing or care resources.

The population consisted of 60 English-speaking dyads of 60 caregivers and their 60 care recipients living in the midwestern United States. There were slightly more African American dyads than Caucasian. Commonality between care receivers was chronic disease and the need for caregiving to maintain living in their homes. Two interviewers simultaneously conducted semistructured interviews with care receivers and caregivers concerning their care experiences using the Relational-Based Joint Decision-Making Model.

Results/Findings: Indications from this study show many aspects of processes in which caregivers and care receivers negotiate the rules or parameters of care dyads; failure to establish them may result in increased caregiver strain. Negotiating was significant in dyadic care relationships, and evidence was found that negotiation skills were needed to enhance interactions. More research is needed to examine the relationship between dyadic negotiation and rules and clinical outcomes.

Implications for Nurses: Nurses play pivotal roles in helping clients and families cope with stressful situations by enhancing communication and interpersonal relationships. Negotiation is a powerful tool that can be used to establish dyadic rules, strengthen relationships, and facilitate positive clinical outcomes.

REFERENCES

Antai-Otong, D. (2001). Creative stress-management for self-renewal. *Dermatology Nursing, 13,* 31–32, 35–39.

Antai-Otong, D. (2006). Psychiatric patients and ethical issues. In V. D. Lachman (ed). *Applied Ethics in Nursing* (pp. 133–144). New York: Springer Publishing Co.

Bailey, P. H., & Tilley, S. (2002). Storytelling and the interpretation of meaning in qualitative research. *Journal of Advanced Nursing, 38,* 574–583.

Baker, L., Rideout, J., Gertler, P., & Raube, K. (2005). Effect of an Internet-based system for doctor-patient communication in health care spending. *Journal of the American Information Association, 19,* 1–20.

Bates, M. S., Rankin-Hill, L., & Sanchez-Ayendez, M. (1997). The effects of cultural context of health care on treatment of and response to chronic pain and illness. *Social Science Medicine, 45,* 1433–1447.

Begley, C. M., & Glacken, M. (2004). Irish nursing students' changing levels of assertiveness during their pre-registration programme. *Nurse Education Today, 24,* 501–510.

Bennett, M. P., Zeller, J. M., Rosenberg, L., & McCann, J. (2003). The effect of mirth laughter on stress and natural killer cell activity. *Alternative Therapy and Health Medicine, 9,* 38–45.

Branger, P. J., van't Hooft, A., van der Wooden, J. C., Duisterhout, J. S., & van Bemmel, J. H. (1998). Shared care for diabetes: Supporting communication between primary and secondary care. *Medinfo, 9*(part 1), 412–416.

Breslin, S., Greskovich, W., & Turisco, F. (2004). Wireless technology improves nursing workflow and communications. *Computers, Informatics Nursing (CIN), 22,* 275–281.

Ceccio, J., & Ceccio, C. M. (1982). *Effective communication in nursing: Theory and practice.* New York: John Wiley & Sons.

Cook, R. I., Render, M., & Woods, D. D. (2000). Gaps in the continuity of care and progress on patient safety. *British Medical Journal, 320,* 791–794.

Cooper, L. A., Roter, D. L., Johnson, R. L., Ford, D. E., Steinwachs, D. M., & Powe, N. R. (2003). Patient-centered communication, ratings of care, and concordance of patient and physician race. *Annals of Internal Medicine, 139,* 907–915.

Dallas, C. (2004). Family matters: How mothers of adolescent parents experience adolescent pregnancy and parenting. *Public Health Nursing, 21,* 47–53.

de Vries, B., Suedfeld, P., Krell, E., Blando, J. A., & Southard, P. (2005). The Holocaust as a context of telling life stories. *International Journal of Aging and Human Development, 60,* 213–228.

Enns, C. Z. (1997). *Feminist theories and feminist psychotherapies: Origins, themes, and variations.* Binghamton, NY: Haworth.

Erikson, E. (1968). *Identity: Youth and crisis.* New York: W. W. Norton.

Fay, A. (2002). The case against boundaries in psychotherapy. In A. A. Lazarus & O. Zur (Eds.), *Dual Relationships and Psychotherapy* (pp. 146–166). New York: Springer.

Gosbee, J. (1998). Communication among health professionals. *British Medical Journal, 316,* 642.

Grant, R. W., Cagliero, E., Chuch, H. C., & Meigs, J. B. (2005). Internet use among primary care patients with type 2 diabetes: The generation and education gap. *Journal of General Internal Medicine, 20,* 470–473.

Hassed, C. (2001). How humour keeps you well. *Australian Family Physician, 30,* 25–28.

Institute of Medicine. (2001). *Crossing the quality chasm. A new health system for the 21st century.* Washington, DC: National Academy Press.

Jourard, S. M. (1964). *The transparent self.* Princeton, NJ: Van Nostrand.

Koch, T., Marks, J., & Tooke, E. (2001). Evaluating a community nursing service: Listening to the voices of clients with an intellectual disability and/or their proxies. *Journal of Clinical Nursing, 10,* 352–363.

Lin, Y. R., Shiah, I. S., Chang, Y. C., Lai, T. J., Wang, K. Y., & Chou, K. R. (2004). Evaluation of an assertiveness training program on nursing and medical students' assertiveness, self-esteem and interpersonal communication satisfaction. *Nurse Education Today, 24,* 656–665.

Liu, J., Pothiban, L., Lu, Z., & Khamphonsiri, T. (2000). Computer knowledge, attitudes, and skills in nurses in People's Hospital of Beijing Medical University. *Computers in Nursing, 18,* 197–206.

Lobb, E. A., Butow, P. N., Kenny, D. T., & Tattersall, M. H. (1999). Communication prognosis of early breast cancer: Do women understand the language used? *Medical Journal of Australia, 171,* 290–294.

MacDonald, C. M. (2004). A chuckle a day keeps the doctor away: Therapeutic humor and laughter. *Journal of Psychosocial Nursing and Mental Health Services, 42,* 18–25.

Martin, R. A. (2001). Humor, laughter, and physical health: Methodological issues and research findings. *Psychological Bulletin, 127,* 504–519.

McCartan, P. J., & Hargie, O. D. (2004). Assertiveness and caring: Are they compatible? *Journal of Clinical Nursing, 13,* 707–713.

Miller, W. R. (1985). Motivation for treatment: A review with special emphasis on alcoholism. *Psychological Bulletin, 98,* 84–107.

Miller, W. R., & Rollnick, S. (1991). *Motivational interviewing: Preparing people to change addictive behavior.* New York: The Guilford Press.

Shellman, J. (2004). "Nobody ever asked me before": Understanding life experiences of African American elders. *Journal of Transcultural Nursing, 15,* 308–316.

The, A. M., Hak, T., Koeter, G., & van Der Wal, G. (2000). Collusion in doctor-patient communication about imminent death: An ethnographic study. *British Medical Journal, 321,* 1376–1381.

Timmins, F., & McCabe, C. (2005a). How assertive are nurses in the workplace? A preliminary pilot study. *Journal of Nursing Management, 13,* 61–67.

Timmins, F., & McCabe, C. (2005b). Nurses' and midwives' assertive behaviour in the workplace. *Journal of Advanced Nursing, 51,* 38–45.

Van Walraven, C., Seth, R., & Laupacis, A. (2002). Hospital discharge summaries infrequently get to posthospitalization physicians. *Canadian Family Physicians, 48*, 737–743.

Von Gunten, G. F., Ferris, F. D., & Emanuel, L. L. (2000). The patient-physician relationship. Enduring competency in end-of-life care: Communication and relational skills. *Journal of the American Medical Association, 284*, 3051–3057.

Wooten, P. (1996). Humor: The antidote for stress. *Holistic Nursing Practice, 10*, 49–56.

Yamashita, M., Forchuk, C., & Mound, B. (2005). Nurse case management: Negotiating care together within a developing relationship. *Perspectives in Psychiatric Care, 41*, 62–70.

SELECTED WEB SITES

Administration on Aging—How to Find Help:
http://www.aoa.gov/eldfam/how_to_find/how_to_find.asp

The Association of Telehealth Service Providers: http://www.atsp.org

Combined Health Information Database (CHID)—Citations, abstracts, and availability information for educational materials on a vast number of health-related topics: http://chid.nih.gov

National Black Association for Speech-Language and Hearing (NBASLH): http://www.nbaslh.org

National Institute on Deafness and Other Communication Disorders (NIDCD)—Free publications in Spanish (en Español):
http://www.nidcd.nih.gov/order/pubs_type.asp?type=spanish

National Institute on Deafness and Other Communication Disorders (NIDCD)—What Is Voice? What Is Speech? What Is Language?:
http://www.nidcd.nih.gov/health/voice/whatis_vsl.asp

Chapter Three

Nurse–Client Interactions: Strengthening Care Partnerships

LEARNING OBJECTIVES

Upon completion of this chapter, the reader should be able to:

- Recognize the significance of nurse–client interactions in a changing health care arena

- Analyze the impact of technologies on interpersonal relationships

- Discuss the relevance of self-awareness in nurse–client interactions

- Characterize Peplau's phases of the nurse–client relationship

- Examine the nurse–client relationship across the life span

- Define shared decision making within the context of nurse–client relationships

- Delineate characteristics of client-centered care

- Describe ethical and legal issue in nurse–client relationships
- Describe end-of-life communication with clients and families across the life span

KEY TERMS

Client-centered care—A health care model that integrates client ideas, expectations, beliefs, values, culture, and emotional and social perspectives, while ensuring mutual (nurse–client) participation in a shared decision-making partnership.

Collaboration—The process of working or cooperating with others to achieve a common goal.

Empathy—The capacity to value and understand the feelings and perceptions of others.

Hospice—A model of care designed to provide comfort and support to clients and their families when a life-limiting illness no longer responds to cure-oriented treatments.

Nurse–client relationship—A dynamic and mutually respective interaction whose goal is valuing, understanding, and embracing the client's unique experiences, preferences, concerns, fears, and wishes using an accepting and insightful approach.

Self-awareness—An internal evaluation of self and one's reactions to emotionally charged situations, people, and places. It affords an opportunity to recognize how our attitudes, perceptions, past and present experiences, and relationships frame or distort interactions with others.

Shared decision making—An interactive and dynamic process between the nurse and client that takes into account ethical and legal considerations. Decisions are based on client preferences, health education, the benefits and risks of available choices, client-centered interventions, and mutually agreed upon treatment planning.

Telemedicine—The use of information technology to provide health care and share clinical information from separate geographic locations.

INTRODUCTION

The therapeutic relationship is a concept that is essential to nursing and the art of healing. Nursing occurs within the context of the nurse–client relationship. The quality, content, and integrity of interpersonal relationships must be nurtured because of their importance to both the nurse and the client. Studies show that effective communication between providers and clients reduces malpractice suits, improves treatment adherence, and leads to positive clinical outcomes (Levinson, Roter, Mulloly, Dull, & Frankel, 1997; Stewart, 1996; Stewart et al., 1999).

The nurse's capacity to form interpersonal relationships is fundamentally important; these relationships evolve from the interplay of verbal and nonverbal negotiations, eventually resulting in mutually respectful relationships (Morse, 1991). Only by knowing our clients can we fully comprehend the meaning of their experiences and appropriately respond to their needs. Factors associated with knowing the client include empathy, trust, respect, and understanding. Self-awareness also is a critical element of valuing the needs of others as well as yourself. Nurses must be considerate and benevolent in caring for clients. Caring requires genuine interest in the client as an individual within the social context of humanity and moral consciousness that preserves dignity and respect (Eriksson, 2002).

Healing relationships are grounded in empathy. **Empathy** enables the nurse to understand inner experiences and communicate them verbally and nonverbally. It is communicated through acceptance, a willingness to listen, and competence to balance personal perspectives with the client's, and it is sustained by maintaining a degree of detachment to ensure a healthy relationship (Katz, 1963). Through empathy, understanding, observation, and sharing the nurse gains perspective about the client's experience, evaluates symptoms, and provides client-centered interventions. Mounting evidence demonstrates the value of empathy in strengthening interpersonal relationships, although there is a lack of agreement about its definition (Stephan & Finlay, 1999). This nurse–client interactive process focuses the nurse's attention on the feelings and experiences of the client. It humanizes nurse–client interactions and enables the nurse to embrace the client's experiences.

Client-centered care refers to a holistic or individualized approach that incorporates client ideas, experiences, wishes, preferences, and cultural, emotional, and social needs while ensuring shared-decision making between the nurse and client. Holistic and client-centered care has been shown to provide higher client satisfaction and more cost-effective and improved clinical outcomes (Donadio, 2005; Wanzer, Booth-Butterfield, & Gruber, 2004).

The integrity of nurse–client interactions is being challenged by rapid changes in health care, an aging population, changing demographics, dwindling resources, a growing incidence of chronic diseases, advances in information technology (e.g., email, Internet, listservs), and demands to deliver continuity of care (Baker, Mainous, Gray, & Love, 2003; Balint & Shelton, 1996; Gill & Mainous, 1998). It also is threatened by health care organizations that devalue time spent communicating with the client to provide client-centered and quality health care (McCabe, 2004).

Now more than ever, the nurse must advocate for quality time to communicate with the client, navigate complex health care systems, and broker client-centered interventions. In this age of marked changes in health care and telecommunications, nurses must strive to establish and maintain enduring nurse–client relationships, ensure open communication, and provide health promotion and well-being relevant to diverse populations and communities (Collins, Clark, Petersen, & Kressin, 2002; Richardson, 2002). Strong interpersonal relationships allow the nurse to act as intermediary and help the client and family navigate the health care system, understand treatment issues, and participate in client- and family-centered care. Quality nurse–client and caregiver relationships offer a healing environment in which the nurse can identity preferences, wishes, and health care practices; develop shared decision making; encourage autonomy; and implement individualized care. Clients must be encouraged to be active participants in their health care.

Shared decision making is an interactive and dynamic process between the nurse and client that must explicitly distinguish mutual and individual responsibilities and expectations of all involved parties. This partnership is grounded in ethical and legal considerations that are based on understanding the client as a whole person, identifying available treatment options and client preferences, and imparting health education. Identifying the benefits and risks of available choices is also part of the decision-making process (Etchells, Sharpe, Burgess, & Singer, 1996; Fallowfield, Lipkin, & Hall, 1998; Siminoff & Step, 2005).

Evidence-based research consistently links shared decision making to a positive impact on clinical outcomes, adherence to treatment, and client and provider satisfaction with the practice of treating clients with dignity and involving them in their own care (Hamann, Leucht, & Kissling, 2003; Lorig et al., 2001; Stewart et al., 1999). The nurse must continually assess and clarify the client's understanding and preferences concerning this process because they may change during the course of treatment. Ultimately, shared decision making becomes the base of the nurse–client relationship, health education, evidence-based interventions, emotional support, and health promotion.

The foremost aim of this chapter is to discuss the significance of the nurse–client relationship within a rapidly changing health care arena, and its ability to preserve client integrity and respect and facilitate optimal levels of functioning for clients across the life span, while maintaining a healthy work environment for the nurse. The chapter will also discuss shared decision making and client-centered approaches as bases of healthy and therapeutic relationships and an appreciation of individual uniqueness. Because the role of the nurse continues to expand, the chapter also will integrate principles and concepts that establish a firm foundation from which to gain knowledge of human interactions, obtain effective communication skills collaborate with others, enhance personal development, and heighten the self-awareness needed to discourse with clients, families, and colleagues.

THE NURSE–CLIENT RELATIONSHIP

As already mentioned, how the nurse communicates with the client can have a vast impact on client satisfaction, health outcomes, and adherence to treatment. Now more than ever, the **nurse–client relationship** is the heart of nursing care and critical to nurses in all practice settings. This concept stems from Hildegard Peplau's seminal work, *Interpersonal Relations in Nursing* (1952). She describes the nurse–client relationship as "a significant, therapeutic interpersonal process. It functions co-operatively with other human processes that make health possible for individuals and communities" (Peplau, p. 16). Although her contributions were made within the context of psychiatric nursing, they transcend specialties and are an integral part of day-to-day nursing.

Inherent in all nurse–client relationships is dynamic communication, with the goal of valuing and embracing the client's unique experience, preferences, concerns, fears, and wishes using an accepting and insightful approach. Peplau's contributions focused on establishing and maintaining quality nurse–client relationships to appraise each client's experiences, anxiety, and needs regarding his or her illness; engage the client in shared decision making concerning treatment; and then develop and implement effective interventions. Other nursing theorists, such as Roy (1970, 1984) also focused on this aspect of healing relationships. Healing and therapeutic relationships allow the client to express feelings openly and confidently.

Peplau further pointed out the importance of the nurse–client relationship as the primary means of providing nursing care. The nurse enters the client's experience through a window of trust and acceptance. Trust is the cornerstone of the nurse–client relationship. It facilitates a caring dialogue that fosters expression of feelings, thoughts, ideas, needs, and experiences and permits the nurse to determine the client's openness to discussing health information, receptiveness to emotional support and adaptive change, and motivation to adhere to treatment. The nurse intentionally guides this interactive relationship to formulate client-centered interventions (Antai-Otong

& Wasserman, 2003). The nurse also must serve as an intermediary between the client and family and the interdisciplinary team.

Peplau explicates four interlocking yet distinct phases of the nurse–client relationship that serve to identify problems, acquire support, mobilize, and strengthen adaptive processes. The four phases are:

- Orientation
- Identification
- Exploitation
- Resolution

Orientation Phase

The orientation phase is central to the nurse–client relationship and shapes the infrastructure of successive phases. Quality and unhurried approaches during this phase permit the nurse to answer questions, explain medical terminology, promote a sense of security, and obtain client understanding of symptoms and treatment choices. According to Peplau's theory, the client directs the relationship by identifying relevant concerns as the nurse facilitates the process, using encouragement and empathy to explore the client's experiences, concerns, and needs (Martin, Forchuk, Santopinto, & Butcher, 1992). Exploring the client's experiences and emotions strengthens the human dimension of nursing. Moreover, it fosters autonomy, self-efficacy, and self-directedness; promotes therapeutic discourse; and expands healing and recovery (Halpern, 2001). The nurse may use diverse roles—such as resource person, teacher, leader, surrogate, counselor, consultant, mediator, and researcher—to create a healing environment and to advance the movement toward health, competence, and an optimal level of functioning (Peplau, 1991).

Establishing rapport and trust and appreciating the client's experiences, health practices, culture, motivation, preferences, and needs—the infrastructure of client-centered care—evidence mastery of this phase. Changing demographics, such as a growing aging and minority populations, require a greater knowledge of cultural differences, health practices, perceptions of illness and health, disparities among diverse populations, and the unique needs of specific populations. Nurses must advocate for and broker the needs of diverse populations and ensure equitable access to treatment and holistic care. Through a strong nurse–client relationship and an emotional context of caring, the client moves from a period of acute distress and vulnerability to one that fosters a healing environment of hope, optimism, healing, self-efficacy, and recovery. A major challenge for today's nurse is that less time is available to establish quality interactions with the client. Because of time constraints, nurses and other health professionals must immediately develop interpersonal relationships within a shorter time span to establish rapport and trust through the experience. For this reason, it is crucial to use quality communication skills, particularly active listening, to initiate and gather important information, assess symptoms, and implement holistic care. (See Chapter 2 for more information about communication skills.) Less time available makes the quality of time spent with the client invaluable in maintaining healthy nurse–client interactions. The following nurse–client dialogue depicts Peplau's orientation and identification phases.

Mr. Perry, a 50-year-old engineer, is being seen in the urgent care clinic with complaints of dizziness, especially when he bends or moves his head. He is fearful and thinks he has a serious medical problem. His last appointment with his primary care provider was 3 months ago, during which time he was given a clean bill of health.

Nurse: Good morning, Mr. Perry, what's brought you in today?

Client: I really feel bad today. I don't know what's wrong with me. *(Feels he knows the meaning of his symptoms)*

Nurse: What do you mean "bad"?

Client: Every time I pick up things from the floor I feel dizzy and weak.

Nurse: How long have you had problems with dizziness when you pick up things?

Client: About 1 or 2 days, right around the time I stopped taking my medication.

Nurse: What medication?

Client: Sertraline. I was on it for 2 months and felt better so I stopped taking it.

Nurse: You stopped taking it? *(Partial mutual understanding of client's symptoms)*

Client: Yes.

Nurse: What does your provider think about your decision to stop your medication?

Client: I don't know. I know how I felt and didn't need permission to stop it! *(Firm individual understanding about his symptoms)*

Nurse: I understand you felt better, but your provider needs to work with you in coming off the medication to reduce the dizziness.

Client: You mean to tell me the dizziness is from stopping the medication? *(Mutual understanding of possible cause of symptoms)*

Nurse: Yes. I need to discuss this with your provider. Do you mind me calling him now so he can evaluate your dizziness?

Client: Sure. I don't like the dizziness, and whatever it takes to get rid of it I'm willing to try. *(Collaborative approach to problem solving)*

Initially, the client expressed feelings of helplessness, anxiety, and fear generated by his symptoms. During the orientation phase he sought evaluation and treatment within the context of the nurse–client relationships. Through empathy, support, patience, and concern, the nurse created a safe and healing environment that encouraged dialogue and expression of feelings and concerns. Although the client was defensive when asked about informing his provider that he stopped his medication, he was able to sort through his feelings and realize the nurse was there to assist him, not to criticize or minimize his preferences, feelings, and health practices.

Identification Phase

The unique aspect of this phase is its focus on identifying and clarifying goals and enacting shared decision making. During this phase the client identifies with the nurse as a helper whom he can trust and collaborate with to facilitate healing and recovery. Within the social context of the nurse–client relationship the nurse nurtures, encourages, mobilizes physical and emotional resources, and provides tools that promote adaptive behavioral changes. Client education and health-promoting activities are essential elements of this phase. Adaptive behavior changes and necessary resources, such as psychosocial support and health education concerning treatment and healthy lifestyle changes, enrich the client's repertoire of coping skills and sharpen focus on interventions that promote an optimal level of mental and physical health. The nurse must also be cognizant of personal biases and life experiences, which may stymie objectivity and prevent the client from reaching an optimal level of functioning. The nurse also must be mindful of the power and stature the client cedes to him or her during this period. Throughout this phase it is very important for the nurse to collaborate with the client, family, and appropriate staff to ensure individualized health care. Individualized care requires identifying and integrating client needs, wishes, health practices, culture, and age-specific tasks into treatment. These client-centered interventions enrich the nurse–client relationship by reducing anxiety and fears, instilling hope and optimism, bolstering self-esteem and confidence, and advancing recovery. As the client moves from the orientation phase of understanding reasons for seeking help and collaborates with the nurse in a shared decision-making process, he or she is prepared and self-directed to take advantage of treatment options during the exploitation phase.

Exploitation Phase

If the orientation and identification phases go smoothly, the client should be self-assured and confident and may actively participant in his or her plan of care. During this phase the client struggles to balance autonomy and dependence. Adaptive coping behaviors emerge secondary to understanding and using health education and other interventions to cope with present stressors and concerns. Toward the end of this phase, the quality of the nurse–client relationship is strengthened by trust and understanding that optimize health promotion and recovery.

Resolution Phase

According to Peplau (1991), the resolution phase "implies the gradual freeing from identification with helping persons . . . and strengthening the ability to stand more or less alone" (p. 40). Generally speaking, quality nurse–client interactions facilitate adaptive changes that move the client from a state of anxiety, fears, uncertainty, and dependency to one of personal growth, self-efficacy, integrity, independence, and optimal functioning. Resolution frees the client from dependency on the nurse–client relationship, allowing the client to manage his or her own symptoms and quality of life.

Naturally, the success of the client moving through these phases is tenuous, and is based on the nurse's repertoire of communication skills, individual responses, client illness, and stress and coping behaviors.

THE IMPACT OF TECHNOLOGIES ON INTERPERSONAL RELATIONS

The Internet: Nurse–Client Connections

The Internet and other technologies have revolutionized communication and how society functions. They are an integral part of everyday life and continue to impact interpersonal relationships and information systems (Purcell, Wilson, & Delamothe, 2002; Silberg, Lundberg, & Musacchio, 1997). Conservative estimates indicate that between 50% and 80% of adults use the Internet to access health information (Horrigan & Rainie, 2002; Taylor, 2002). These findings indicate that more and more clients are communicating with nurses and other providers via varied technologies including email, monitoring devices, virtual support groups, videoconferencing, interactive voice response (IVR).

Historically, face-to-face contact was perceived as the most effective and expeditious way in which to establish a nurse–client relationship. However, face-to-face contact increasingly has been replaced by electronic technologies that connect clients with nurses and other providers. Growing data indicate clients feel empowered by information acquired from the Internet because it helps communicate their health care needs and concerns more clearly, quickly, and productively via email than face-to-face visits with providers (Lin, Wittevrongel, Moore, Beaty, & Ross, 2005).

Several studies cite the cost-effectiveness and efficiency of email as a means of communication between client and provider; it also is a method of communication that has high client satisfaction (Feldman, Murtaugh, Pezzin, McDonald, & Peng, 2005). Researchers submit that emails actually increased adherence to self-monitoring, promote a sense of self-efficacy in chronic disease management, and reduce the necessity of face-to-face interaction (Lin et al., 2005; Ketteridge, Delbridge, & Delbridge, 2005). In a retrospective study by Ketteridge and colleagues (2005), 306 clients undergoing elective surgery received email health education, compared to 352 in a control group who did not receive email health information. Findings from this study indicated that 16% of those who received email health education used email communication, whereas 3% in the control group used email communication. The researchers concluded that routine health education via email was an effective means of communicating with clients undergoing elective surgery.

Another study involving the Florida Initiative in Telehealth and Education (FITE) diabetes initiative reviewed the opinions of 44 clients, 6 caregivers, 6 case managers, and 18 school nurses, family members, and other providers who took part in an online education project. The study showed that participants expressed satisfaction with the technology and the process, and communication was improved (Malasanos, Patel, Klein, & Burlingame, 2005). Findings from these studies indicate the innovative quality of communicating with client using email and other technologies.

Despite the benefits of the Internet and other electronic messaging systems, ethical and legal concerns exist. Major ethical dilemmas include client privacy, confidentiality, and Web site security. How is the site maintained, and is information disseminated via a secure information system? The privacy of client information is often violated when online information can be accessed by unintended parties or when it is recorded through various means such as IVR, video recording, or data transmission through technologies (Health Information Portability and Accountability Act of 1996 [HIPAA]). Prior to using any form of electronic communication, the nurse must determine if the Web site is secure, who has access to client data, and follow the organization policy on information technology. Personal information transmitted via email or the Internet requires encryption and protection of private data.

Scientists have explored the impact of various technological modalities on human interactions. Although there is a lack of consensus about the impact of various technologies, including email, the telephone, and the Internet, on human relationships, some submit that non-face-to-face contact may result in less personal filtering (e.g., transmission and reception of verbal and nonverbal cues), less predictable responses, miscommunication, more time needed to establish rapport, less opportunities for feedback, and potentially negative consequences for interpersonal relationships (Neuhauser & Kreps, 2003; Riva, 2002). Apart from these barriers associated with e-health communication via vast technologies, literacy, linguistic, cultural, age-related difficulties, and disabilities, as well as a required higher reading levels on the Web, pose an even greater problem for about 50% of the United States population (Eysenbach & Jadad, 2001). Despite potential barriers to establishing rapport and potential negative consequences of the Internet, email, and other technologies, there is growing reliance and evidence of positive outcomes using vast technologies to communicate with and treat clients who prefer to receive health care in their homes and community settings.

Overall, the Internet and email have revolutionized communication and created a host of opportunities for nurse–client dialogues, dissemination of health education, emotional support, and client-centered care. One aspect of distance technology, telemedicine, shows great promise in delivering health care in the client's home and increasing access to health care.

Telemedicine

More and more people live in remote and underserved areas, making it difficult for clients to travel to primary care and other settings to access health care. Distant travel is particularly burdensome to frail older adults and their caregivers. As more and more clients become computer literate and have computers in their homes, nurses are in a pivotal position to ensure these clients' linkage with health care through meaningful nurse–client relationships.

The Institute of Medicine (IOM) has suggested the use of information technologies and electronic medical records (EMR) as a means of securing quality care, efficiency, and client safety (IOM, 2001). Recommendations from the IOM continue to be integrated into health care systems. One example of health care's transition to computer applications and client data management is telemedicine.

Telemedicine is information technology employed to provide health care and share clinical information between two geographic locations (Rafiq & Merrell, 2005). Telemonitoring technologies are being used to monitor clients in their homes. Several studies have shown the efficiency of a specific home-telehealth strategy for care coordination intended to improve functional independence in noninstitutionalized veterans with chronic disease (Chumbler, Mann, Wu, Schmid, & Kobb, 2004). Care coordination home telehealth (CCHT) has proven especially effective for individuals living in remote or underserved areas managing chronic diseases and for whom traveling is burdensome. CCHT affords daily nurse–client interaction through telemonitoring equipment. Although this system does not provide face-to-face contact, it offers reassurance and confidence that the clients are "connected" with the nurse. Through daily interaction, the nurse is able to monitor and manage symptoms, although they are self-reported in some cases; provide emotional support and early problem identification; make just-in-time referrals to urgent or emergency care; and provide health education. Initial contact with these clients occurs in primary clinics or other medical settings or in the home, where the nurse assesses the client's ability to comprehend and manage the equipment. Caregivers are also included in the decision-making process. Trust, rapport, and ultimately the nurse–client relationship evolve from initial contact and endure throughout treatment. Daily contact enables the nurse to monitor signs and symptoms using chronic disease parameters and foster self-care management and adherence to treatment. Daily entries from blood pressure monitors, scales, and glucometers, as well as physical symptoms are monitored. In the event the client fails to enter data for several days, or if the nurse is concerned about the client's condition, a telephone call is used to check on the client, provide health education, and make health care decisions (Chumbler et al., 2004). Continual monitoring helps many clients feel safe and secure, knowing the nurse is a telephone call away. CCHT also has proven to be cost-effective, improve client satisfaction, and reduce resource utilization secondary to decreased emergency room visits and hospitalizations.

Internet technologies continue to transform how nurses communicate with their clients. They link the nurse to the client, thus improving access to health care, expanding client participation in their own care, enhancing health education and adherence to treatment, and facilitating shared decision making. Despite these advantages, electronic technologies cannot replace the fundamental and human aspects of face-to-face contact, which is the foundation of nurse–client relationships. Face-to-face contact is optimal for providing meaningful care, making accurate diagnoses based on direct observation of verbal and nonverbal cues, and promoting comfort through human contact.

Although technological advances are available to many, a large number of clients living in poverty and in remote and rural areas lack access to various telecommunication methods. Predictably, a lack of access to technologies contributes to health disparities, limits access to health care, and contributes to poor clinical outcomes. Solutions to this problem are complex and require innovative strategies such as community outreach, involvement in client advocacy groups, and legislative action. An extensive discussion of health disparities and potential solutions involving communication is provided in Chapter 4, Cultural Aspects of Communication Partnerships.

More research is needed to develop telecommunication processes that ensure client privacy and confidentiality, cost-effectiveness, and client satisfaction. Efforts must also be made to develop technologies that link diverse cultural, multilingual, and socioeconomic populations to health care and facilitate appropriate access to health care the client needs. The expansion in communication technology continues to have a profound impact on the nurse–client relationship and nursing practice. However, nurses still must establish quality communication with clients and their families across the health care continuum and maintain processes that sustain these relationships.

SELF-AWARENESS AND PERSONAL DEVELOPMENT

As mentioned already in this chapter, healthy nurse–client relationships create a climate of mutual trust and respect. Fundamental to this relationship is an awareness of how the nurse contributes to or diminishes mutual trust. The first step to understanding how we relate to and discourse with others is tuning in to ourselves through self-awareness.

Meier and her colleagues (2001) describe **self-awareness** as a professional obligation when caring for the ill because it may mitigate distress, burnout, and poor clinical judgment. Self-awareness is an internal evaluation of yourself and your reaction to intense emotional situations, people, and places. It helps the nurse recognize how her or his attitudes, perceptions, past and present experiences, and relationships frame or distort interactions with others and their potential impact on interpersonal relationships. Recognizing these issues is crucial to reducing biases, stereotyping, and inappropriate or negative reactions (Antai-Otong & Wasserman, 2003).

One area in which self-awareness is especially important is working with clients who are seriously ill or who have end-of-life conditions. Strong client emotions can impede nurse–client communication. Predictably, a client's emotional reactions tend to generate similar emotions in the nurse. Moreover, the nurse's past experiences with death and dying; his or her coping skills, values, beliefs, and health practices; and the nature of his or her relationship with the client govern the nurse's emotional and behavioral responses to given situations. Common emotional reactions range from a need to rescue to a sense of failure or guilt and frustration, a feeling of powerlessness, and a fear of becoming ill. Intense emotional reactions are uncomfortable and can make the nurse want to avoid the client and separate him- or herself from end-of-life situations. Under these circumstances, self-awareness can guide internal self-monitoring and help the nurse appraise how feelings and strong emotions govern the way he or she listens, perceives, and reacts to the client and others. Self-awareness also expands personal strengths and provides insight regarding personal limitations. Recognizing your personal responses to clients is the first step to controlling them. Nurses must realize that emotional reactions are normal, but the degree to which they impact nurse–client relationships must be examined so they do not distort objective data collection, diagnosis, and goal setting, or disrupt the therapeutic environment. Strategies nurses can use in response to end-of-life and other stressful circumstances include the following:

- Recognize emotional and behavioral responses.
- Acknowledge the normalcy of these reactions.
- Examine the reasons for these personal reactions and the potentially adverse consequences of them.

• Discuss these feelings and thoughts with a friend or family member (Antai-Otong & Wasserman, 2003; Epstein, 1999; Grunfeld et al., 2000; Novack et al., 1997; Jenkins & Elliott, 2004).

(See Chapters 1 and 2 for a lengthy discussion on self-awareness as a personal growth tool.)

Lack of self-awareness or poor insight into personal responses hinders the communication process, engenders distrust, and compromises health care. More significantly, it destroys trust and impedes opportunities to understand the client's experiences, needs, and values, and frequently results in inappropriate treatment planning and negative clinical outcomes. Often, the only indication of poor insight is when the client responds with nonverbal or verbal cues that convey negative responses or evoke strong emotional reactions. In the event a client expresses anger or distrust about your intentions to help, evaluate how you communicated the message to ensure your verbal and nonverbal cues sent a congruent message. Of course, some clients are easily upset because they feel helpless and angry and project negative feelings on the nurse. In these situations, it is necessary to provide a supportive and unbiased response to reduce anxiety and facilitate therapeutic interfaces. Avoid personalizing or sharing negative reactions because they jeopardize trust and effective communication. Again, acknowledging your reactions to different situations, clients, and people strengthens self-awareness and appreciation of others' experiences and perspectives.

Obviously, quality nurse–client relationships are influenced by a variety of factors including self-awareness, life experiences, culture, ethnicity, and developmental issues. The next section integrates the nurse–client relationship and communication patterns across the life span by emphasizing tasks unique to each developmental stage, from infancy to older adulthood.

LIFE SPAN CONSIDERATIONS

Knowledge of normal age-related physical, psychosocial, and development changes is crucial when working with all age groups—infants, toddlers, children, adolescents, adults, and older adults. Understanding these variables can guide the nursing process and promote the use of effective and age-appropriate communication skills. Transactions between individuals across the life span require basic knowledge of biologic, developmental, psychosocial, cultural, and spiritual influences that shape communication patterns and interpersonal relationships. Nurses must actively establish and employ interpersonal relationships as a venue to foster trust, growth and development, and integrity; further health promotion; and strengthen coping and communication skills across the life span.

Infancy and Childhood

Initial sensory experiences mold lifelong learning within a social and cultural context that governs speech patterns, behavior, cognition, and self-concept, and gives meaning to verbal and nonverbal cues and communication patterns over time. Through communication people learn to express feelings, relate to others, clarify problems, gain support, transmit and receive information, and garner a perspective of themselves, the world, and the future.

One of the earliest forms of communication for infants is touch or tactile sensory stimulation. It is well established that even during the neonatal period, touch and various forms of communication are essential for survival. Early parental touching, bathing, and stroking may have a positive impact on developmental mastery as well as mental and physical development (Messmer et al., 1997; Phillips & Moses, 1996). Roy & Andrews (1999) submits that touch is essential for survival, even during gestation, and sensory stimulation modulates and expands crucial biological, psychological, and social processes necessary for survival and adaptation. Early sensory stimulation and communication influence one's self-concept, self-esteem, and ability to form and maintain meaningful relationships, and sustains health and coping patterns over time. Health is defined as "a process and state of being, and becoming whole and integrated in a way that reflects person and environment mutuality" (Roy & Andrews, 1999, p. 19).

In *Interpersonal Relations in Nursing*, Peplau (1952) asserts that external factors influence human development across the life span. Within the social context, the infant assimilates the attitudes and customs of a given society and culture, which become the foundation of lifelong biological, social, and interpersonal development. Nurses caring for infants, children, and their families are challenged to work with individuals within a social and family context governed by diverse and complex factors. Families share the same goal of restoration and healing and must be enlisted in the collaborative process to reach optimal treatment goals.

Hospitalized and critically ill children and their parents are exposed to numerous stressors, which heighten vulnerability to considerable acute and prolonged adverse emotional, behavioral, and academic consequences (Melnyk, Alpert-Gillis, Hensel, Cable-Billing, & Rubenstein, 1997). Nurses must distinguish between normal and abnormal responses in the child and parents and initiate interventions to help them adapt to stressful situations (Melnyk, Alpert-Gillis, Feinstein et al., 2004). The nurse–client relationship is crucial to health promotion and mobilizing adaptive coping responses. Empirical data indicate the importance of involving parents in the care of acutely or chronically ill children (Melnyk, Alpert-Gillis, Feinstein et al., 2004; Roden, 2005). In addition, knowledge of normal responses to end-of-life illnesses enables the nurse to support the youth and parents and facilitate shared decision making.

A randomized, controlled trial with posthospitalization follow-up assessment was conducted with 174 mothers and their young children who were unexpectedly hospitalized in pediatric ICU. Melnyk and her colleagues (2004) found that mothers who participated in the Creating Opportunities for Parent Empowerment (COPE) model program demonstrated improved maternal function and coped more effectively compared to those who did not participate, and subsequently the children coped more effectively with the situation and had fewer emotional and behavioral problems (Melnyk Alpert-Gillis, Feinstein et al., 2004). (See Research Study 3-1 on page 143.)

Failing to collaborate with the client and parents results in interpersonal tension, conflicts, and mistrust and causes enormous stress to both the child and his or her parents. Nurses must create a caring and warm environment that promotes a sense of security and assists in expression of feelings. Communication problems with the nurse and other staff aggravate parental stress. In an exploratory qualitative study of 14 in-depth interviews involving parents and nurses in the care of acutely ill children in Australia, content analysis demonstrated four major themes emerged from interviews with parents: control, emotional support, communication, and the significance of being with their child (Roden, 2005). The mothers also wanted to "do the mothering" and have the nurses "do the nursing." Content analysis also confirmed poor nurse–parent interpersonal relationships as a barrier to quality and healing nurse–client relationships. Major implications from these findings were a need to strengthen nurse–parent communications through workshops and to add training to university curriculum as a pediatric elective (Roden). Data from this study validate Melnyk and colleagues' (2004) findings and emphasize the importance of quality nurse–parent interactions and that interventions are necessary to empower parents and their children.

It is crucial for nurses to assess each family's unique concerns; anxiety level; preferences; wishes; psychosocial, cultural, and spiritual factors; and health practices. Control of one's daily life and child's health is particularly important during stressful times; this is even more relevant for parents with sick children. The child's comfort and healing are mediated by the parents' level of stress and adaptive coping responses.

Adolescence

Working with adolescents requires knowledge about this age group's unique developmental tasks and motivation. The developmental stage of adolescence is marked by the normal growth and development of secondary sex characteristics. During this period the youth becomes increasingly aware of self-image, and is confronted with issues such as intimacy, acceptance by schoolmates, sexuality, and identity. Adolescents and their families struggle with developmental challenges involving rebelliousness and independence. The struggles of adolescence inherent during this developmental period can be enriching and are necessary for the transition from youth to adulthood.

Communicating with adolescents is critical during stressful situations. Nurse–client interactions may be strained by the need to ensure privacy, establish trust, and maintain clear and distinct boundaries. Frequently, adolescents are reluctant to share personal information with nurses and other health care professionals, particularly personal issues such as sexuality and birth control, for fear of this information being shared with parents. Nurses must be honest and open about privacy concerns and information that must be shared with their parents, such as danger to self or others.

Medical and psychiatric problems further challenge the adolescent and parents to adapt to the changes associated with adolescence, and increase the risk of negative emotional, psychosocial, self-image, and academic outcomes. Similar to working with critically ill or hospitalized children and their parents, the nurse must understand the developmental task of adolescence and assess emotional and behavioral problems associated with ineffective coping. The nurse must establish rapport with the youth and parents and enlist them in collaborative relationships that facilitate self-efficacy and health promotion. Health education programs for the self-management of various medical conditions in adolescents and their families have demonstrated reduced health care costs, lowered morbidity, and improved self-efficacy. The nurse must tailor treatment consistent with the adolescent's cultural and spiritual needs; unique circumstances; and motivation to improve knowledge, skills, self-image, while also enhancing her or his sense of control and self-esteem.

Families

Children exist within the social context of families. Family values, beliefs, ethnicity, culture, communication patterns, health practices, adaptive coping behaviors, and methods of communication are instilled through family interactions across the life span. Ideally, early family interactions and social contexts are positive, engaging, and enriching, and form the basis for mutual respect and acceptance, open and honest communication, altruism, individual achievement or actualization, and independence.

Children spend most of their time with families who meet their basic human needs, provide socialization, teach them how to communicate, share values, and provide an environment of love, acceptance, and companionship. Because of the vast diversity among families, it behooves nurses working with infants, children, and adolescents to assess and identify the family's uniqueness. Socioeconomic status and educational preparation also influence children's health and their ability to maximize strengths during crisis and noncrisis situations. Over the past decade a greater emphasis on family-centered care has been successfully advocated. This concept is especially relevant to establishing open and quality communication among the nurse, children, and families, particularly when the child is hospitalized and the family faces enormous stress. During stressful periods, knowledge of family dynamics may help the nurse assist the client in resolving current and past interpersonal discord.

A family stress model created by Conger and colleagues (2000) depicts stress as the basis of parent and emotional distress and marital instability that disrupts parenting and the quality of parent–child interactions, and can cause short-term or enduring poor outcomes. Disruptive communication between children and their families often manifests as behavioral problems and worsening physical symptoms. Early identification of these behaviors and evidence of family discord must be addressed. Referrals for family or marital therapy must be considered when strife has a negative impact on the child and family. Prior to making these referrals, concerns need to be discussed with the interdisciplinary team to determine appropriate interventions.

Families are the most lasting social context for children, and the family's health is inextricably tied to the child's health and well-being. Clearly, establishing nurse–client interactions with the family and child are critical to shared decision making and the child's care.

Middle Adulthood

Middle adulthood challenges individuals to take a look at their lives and gain control over the present and future. Because of normal physiological changes middle-aged individuals experience changed vision, hearing, and a slowed down metabolism and sexual function. Middle-aged individuals seek to maintain control of their lives and bodies to maintain emotional and physical integrity. Communication is particularly important to meet personal needs, maintain control over one's life, and to explore the meaning of one's life. Medical conditions, especially serious or debilitating illnesses, may engender feelings of helplessness and loss of control. Although, these feelings are not unique to this age group, it is of particular significance during a period when people take stock of their lives and plan for retirement.

Feelings of helplessness can be mitigated through shared decision making and health education, which the nurses facilitate a sense of empowerment and control. Adults in this age group are often caring for their adult children and for their aging parents. It is imperative to assess the quality of social support systems and involve them in the decision-making process when the client seeks treatment for medical or psychiatric conditions. Caring for serious mentally or physically ill clients and their families is a growing concern across all health care systems. Efforts to provide quality and client-centered care are primary goals that facilitate an optimal level of functioning, mental and physical comfort, and health and quality lifestyles. Although information in this section extends to other age groups across the life span, the emphasis provides general communication issues experienced by individuals in this population.

Older Adulthood

As life expectancies rise, most nurses will be involved in caring for older adults. As with other age groups, the nurse must be able to establish effective communication and interpersonal interactions with individuals 65 and older. Common age-related issues that impact communication include decreased hearing and vision, cognitive changes caused by medical and psychiatric conditions, and polypharmacy. Although each older adult must be assessed and treated individually, it is crucial to assess for these changes and implement interventions that maximize the client's strengths and abilities, maintain collateral communication with caregivers, and assure comfort, a sense of security, integrity, respect, and dignity.

Older adults, like other age groups, depend on communication to relate to others within a caring and compassionate environment based on culture and ethnicity, personal life experiences, respect, and dignity. Special cultural and age-related issues must be carefully assessed and integrated into holistic treatment planning. Ageism is frequently a concern when working with older adults and must be avoided to reduce stereotyping or bias. Each older adult brings a story and repertoire of unique experiences, and when queried will usually share these with the nurse. Storytelling is a powerful tool that enhances the assessment process. It enables the nurse to enter the client's lifelong and present experiences. Knowledge of these experiences provides a resource for client-centered care. Paying careful attention, using patience, and being respectful are necessary communication skills that help the nurse establish meaningful and trusting relationships, which helps improve the client's quality of life (Bowers, Esmond, & Jacobson, 2000) and enhance job satisfaction in caregivers (Rundqvist & Severinsson, 1999). Researchers continue to confirm these tenets. In a study conducted by McGilton and colleagues (2003) using a relationship-enhancing program of care (REP), the researchers concluded that a REP of care for residents living in extended-care facilities enhanced relational skills between residents and nursing staff and improved residents' perceptions of their caregivers and their behavior.

In addition to the client, the nurse also must pursue and establish relationships with families and caregivers to obtain and sometimes validate accurate information concerning health status, personal needs, health practices, and quality of support systems (See Research Study 3-2 on page 144.) Sensory and cognitive deficits and speech difficulties must be assessed to determine the degree to which they impact the client's ability to communicate and participate in decision making. Medical conditions such as strokes often impede information processing or slow down understanding. This is particularly evident in clients experiencing end-of-life situations. Using simple questions and clear sentences, explaining all procedures and treatment, speaking slowly, facing the client with eye contact, and using therapeutic touch are communication methods that facilitate nurse– client transactions and provide reassurance and comfort.

Older adults often view nursing homes and hospitals as places to die. It is essential to communicate with the client and family, provide pragmatic reassurance and hope about death and dying issues, and listen to their stories to assess the meaning of present experiences, fears, and anxieties. This process is enhanced when the nurse initiates and sustains communication with interdisciplinary team members and acts as an intermediary between staff and older adults and their families.

COLLABORATIVE RELATIONSHIPS

The Client and Family

Collaboration is the process of working or cooperating with others to achieve a common goal. Collaboration assumes all sides can win or benefit, and although everyone's needs may not be met, maintaining the interpersonal relationship is worthwhile and necessary to advance individual goals. In other words, the nurse and client have a sense of ownership and investment because of mutual commitment to shared decision making and goal attainment. Shared decision making must parallel evidence-based practice with a focus on the client's unique circumstances, expectations, fears, needs, health practices, values, culture, ethnicity, and capabilities (Stewart et al., 1999). Clients and their families need to comprehend specific procedures, relevant treatment issues, informed consent, and health education, whether they opt to participate in the shared decision-making process or not (Elwyn, Edwards, Kinnersley, & Grol, 2000; Sullivan, 2003). The following points are critical to ensuring quality nurse–client collaboration and resolving communication challenges:

- Allot adequate time to form rapport and trust.
- Exhibit a readiness to understand the client's concerns.
- Impart empathy and respect.
- Affirm commitment to the client's best interests, choices, preferences, and needs.
- Encourage active participation in shared decision making, including options in care.
- Negotiate differences in perspectives.
- Make shared decisions that are palatable to clients, families, the nurse, and the interdisciplinary team. (Antai-Otong & Wasserman, 2003; Harms et al., 2004; Roter, et al., 1997)

The following scenario illustrates a collaborative dialogue between the nurse and a young adult who has just been diagnosed with insulin-dependent diabetes:

Nurse: Good morning, Mark.

Client: What's so good about this morning? I'm diabetic and I'm really freaked out about it.

Nurse: What frightens you the most about having diabetes?

Client: Knowing that I have to give myself a shot every morning. I hate needles!

> **Nurse:** I know having diabetes and giving yourself injections every day is pretty scary. Most people feel this way when they are diagnosed with insulin-dependent diabetes.
>
> **Client:** I'm *not* everybody. I've always eaten what I wanted and now I have to go on a special diet.
>
> **Nurse:** Well, you certainly know what you need to do to control your diabetes. It sounds like the scariest part of all of this is giving yourself insulin injections.
>
> **Client:** Yeah, you're right. My grandmother had diabetes and she had to take shots, too.
>
> **Nurse:** Your grandmother also had diabetes? How did she do?
>
> **Client:** She did alright. In fact, it didn't slow her down at all.
>
> **Nurse:** So what does this tell you about having diabetes?
>
> **Client:** I'm still scared of needles, but if she could do it, I can try.
>
> **Nurse:** Alright! It takes a lot of willpower to stay on track, but I have confidence in you. Let's begin by learning how to give yourself insulin injections.

This scenario demonstrates the importance of sharing information and feelings and exploring options to manage a stressful and scary situation. The nurse facilitated the shared decision-making process, which necessitated active listening with genuine interest, patience, open-ended questioning, and a willingness to focus on the client's world and convey empathy by acknowledging the normalcy of his fears. She also used information about his grandmother to demonstrate how people learn to cope with medical problems and maintain control over their lives.

The Interdisciplinary Team

Quality health care requires a system or interdisciplinary team approach rather than individual efforts. One of the benefits of interdisciplinary teams is the ability to maximize the resources and talents of various disciplines to ensure comprehensive and interactive evidence-based health care (American Hospital Association Commission on Workforce for Hospitals and Health

System, 2002). A collaborative effort among various health care professionals involves shared decision making with a focus on client-centered health care and advancing and integrating safe and quality treatment.

Various services within and outside the health care arena also require collaboration. As when working with clients and families, collaboration with staff requires a clear and professional interface that ensures client confidentiality, accurate information sharing, both written documentation and verbal interactions, and appropriate allocation of resources. It also requires a clear understanding of each team member's role, unique contributions, and responsibilities to ensure appropriate resource allocation, productive discussions, and a holistic plan of care. Reaching a consensus about roles and responsibilities requires strong communication and negotiating skills. An effective team member must also embrace others' personal attributes and respect the rights of others. Getting nurses and other staff to agree on strategies to pursue and attain these goals is fraught with tension, conflicts, differences of opinion, and frustration. During these potentially heated conversations the nurse must be assertive and use active listening, negotiation, and conflict management skills to maintain quality communication and make clinical decisions that ensure quality and safe health care. Obviously, ineffective communication and a failure to resolve conflicts and disagreements between the nurse and staff have potentially negative consequences, including diminished trust, decreased staff morale, staff frustration, anger, dissatisfaction, reduced productivity, and less effective client outcomes.

More and more health care decisions require collaborative processes to ensure quality and safe health care. Ethical and legal considerations are critical components of these processes. The next section focuses on ethical and legal dilemmas regarding telecommunication technologies, confidentiality and privacy, advanced directives, and end of life.

ETHICAL AND LEGAL CONSIDERATIONS

You've Got Email: Benefits and Liabilities

Online communication has the capacity to increase access to care, promote client involvement in their own care, improve outcomes, and reduce health care costs. *Interactive health communication* involves the consumer, client, caregiver, or professional using electronic technologies to "access or transmit health information or receive guidance on a health-related issue [i.e., telemedicine]" (Eng, 2001). Although this approach seems like a logical extension of the nurse–client relationship, it raises legal and ethical concerns. Some researchers assert that electronic client–clinician communication may disrupt the balances in that relationship and create wider gaps in clinical status outcomes for different segments of the population (Hamvas et al., 1996) and impede access to health care (Mandl, Kohane, & Brandt, 1998). Despite these concerns, most research indicates that email and other electronic technologies can enhance nurse–client relationships if implementation strategies are planned ahead of time to ensure secure channels for health communication sites and maintain confidentiality and client privacy consistent with HIPAA and other regulatory guidelines.

Nurse–client transactions involving email may be more effective and practical when a quality relationship already exists. Prior to establishing email or other Internet nurse–client transactions, certain parameters must be established to negotiate boundaries; ensure privacy and informed consent; specify the limitations of the relationship, response times, and subject matter; and determine message or information storage and management methods (Eysenbach & Diepgen, 1999; Spielberg, 1999). Another benefit of email is that it is a very efficient method of communication, particularly when the nurse uses it to provide test results, give information about the next appointment, impart health education, follow up on data obtained from home monitoring devices, or consult with clients or refer them to specialty clinics.

As already discussed, questions concerning security and the nurse's duty of confidentiality remain a concern. Historically, information was maintained in written records and stored in a relatively secure medical records department. With more and more facilities using computerized client records to increase provider efficiency, facilitate easy access to client records, and ensure care across the continuum, the risk of breaching privacy and confidentiality increases. Technology also allows diverse entities, such as payers and consulting staff, to access this information, further jeopardizing confidentiality (Gostin, 2001). Presently there are no formal legal parameters regarding how to maintain the confidentiality and privacy of client medical records, despite concerns raised by the Supreme Court (*Whalen v. United States*, 429 US 589 [1966]).

Online technologies also require collaboration with information technology and facility staff to develop policies and training to ensure appropriate firewalls, Web security, and encryption so that client records are kept confidential.

Advance Directive Planning

Another topic of interest is advance directive planning or end-of-life decisions. Although the Patient Self-Determination Act and Cruzan decision by the Supreme Court suggested the client has the ability to make difficult deci-sions at the end of life, they failed to delineate a provision to implement these ideas (Sullivan, 2002). Recent headlines concerning the Terri Schiavo, right to "live or die," case in Florida point out how tenuous or insufficient signed or verbal agreements can be for enforcing the wishes of loved ones and at end of life. Prior to this case, most people had a misperception that advance direc-tives ensured or protected the client and family's wishes concerning quality of life and unwanted life support measures when the integrity of life was threat-ened. Realistically, the courts appear to view each decision individually and based on factors, including political climate or media awareness, the client and family's wishes concerning end-of-life issues may not be observed.

A subject that is often under discussed is how to communicate with clients and families facing end-of-life issues. A nurse may avoid this subject because of her or his personal reactions, or she or he may avoid or minimize the issue because it engenders strong emotions and personal reactions to death and dying issues. It is ethically sound and vital to recognize death as part of the life span, respect client autonomy, and afford the client and family opportunities to grieve, mourn, express feelings, decide on treatment options, and come to terms and resolve end-of-life issues.

END-OF-LIFE COMMUNICATION

Palliative Care

Advance directives are particularly relevant to nurses providing palliative care. Larson & Tobin (2000) describe advance care planning for the dying client as an element in a series of continuous communications that collec-tively help the client approach death with dignity while respecting personal values, beliefs, culture, and wishes. Currently, no data show that advance directives significantly facilitate decision making, direct care, or are cost-effective at the end of life (Morrison et al., 2005; Teno, Fisher et al., 2000). Many clients and their families struggling with life or death issues generate their choices based on interpersonal relationships and after communication with their physician and members of the health care team. Converging data indicate the importance of quality, effective communication about end-of-life decision making (Field & Cassel, 1997; Fins et al., 1999). Barriers to such communication are vast and include hesitancy on the part of the nurse and other health care professionals (Heaven & Macguire, 1997; Jarrett & Payne,

1995) as well as clients and their families (Hinton, 1998). Clients and families often avoid these dialogues because of cultural and religious factors and the stigma associated with specific health problems (Blackhall, Murphy, Frank, Michel, & Azen, 1995), denial, shyness (Tobin, 1999), and fears of death and dying and the ultimate prognosis.

Tulsky (2005) suggests using the following key aspects of communication with the client and family to engender quality relationships, offer a venue for empathy and responding to the client and family's emotional needs, focus on client-centered goals, and provide minimal attention to specific interventions:

- Create a climate that encourages the client and family to express and share their thoughts and feelings.
- Communicate a consistent message and avoid criticizing other health care providers.
- Appreciate the client's concerns, fears, and anxiety.
- Admit shortcomings or mistakes.
- Remain unassuming.
- Convey empathy, respect, and compassion.
- Allow time to consider and make decisions. (Tulsky, 2005)

The next section focuses on death and dying issues, with a particular focus on communicating with the dying or seriously ill patient of any age. Knowing what to say and how to talk to someone who is dying is challenging to most people. It is crucial for the student, novice, and experienced nurse to communicate with the dying client to ensure dignity and respect. This process begins with embracing your own feelings and thoughts about death and dying. As previously discussed, self-awareness is an integral part of effective nurse–client interactions dealing with stressful or difficult client situations.

The Dying or Seriously Ill Child or Adolescent

The imminent or eventual death of a child is conceivably the worst heartbreak a family ever has to bear. A report from the IOM pointed out the necessity to address challenges associated with the care of dying youths and their parents (Committee on Palliative End-of-Life Care, 2003). Most nurses feel ill-prepared to communicate with children and families confronted with end-of-life situations, or even to cope with their own personal reactions.

Early in his or her career, each nurse needs to concede the difficulties involved with working with seriously ill youth and how it may impede honest communication. The communication that occurs among children, parents, the nurse, and members of the interdisciplinary health team at the end of the youth's life must be grounded in sensitivity, empathy, and compassionate relationships. These relationships require special skills, knowledge, and attitudes that should be fully adopted by the interdisciplinary team. The interdisciplinary approach integrates medical management and optimizes psychosocial, spiritual, and emotional well-being (Wolfe, Friebert, & Hilden, 2002). Frequently the nurse acts as an intermediary between the interdisciplinary team and the client and his or her family members. The nurse's special presence in this process promotes a sense of security for both the youth and the family and helps the nurse garner a sense of their response to their end-of-life experience.

An interdisplinary approach must also center on the youth's, parents', and family's needs and preferences. Converging data indicate that terminally ill children benefit from opportunities to talk about their eventual death (Hilden et al., 2001; Masera et al., 1999). Honest and compassionate communication without subduing hope is pivotal in providing holistic care to the child and family while mitigating uncertainties. Any hope afforded must be pragmatic and pertinent. Major barriers to establishing nurse–client relationships with seriously ill children include poor communication and interpersonal skills, families' unrealistic expectations of medical care, the tremendous emotional burden on the parents, and psychosocial and cultural factors (Faulkner, 1997; Liben, 1996). Nurses must begin a dialogue with the child or adolescent and his or her family to create healing and supportive interactions while encouraging them that they will endure this uncertainty and loss of control as a family unit.

It is important for the nurse to assess the parents' perspective about sharing medical information with the child and clarify the advantages of balancing disclosure and the parents' natural need to protect the child. Discussions among the nurse, child, and family must be guided by the child's intellectual and emotional maturity. A willingness to talk to the child and parents increases shared decision making, mitigates anxiety, promotes comfort, and lightens the burden of secrecy, issues that generate family tension concerning the child's eventual death (Beale, Baile, & Aaron, 2005; Davies, Steele, Collins, Cook, & Smith, 2004). Parents and family members provide invaluable insight into their expectations, observations, values, beliefs, and perceptions regarding the end-of-life experience. The plan of care for the dying child must integrate respect for the dignity of the child and family, including siblings, regarding diagnostic tests, observations, and treatment responses. Respect the child and family's spiritual and cultural needs. Prayers and other spiritual and religious rituals, such as referencing God or making other religious statements, are comforting and often used to cope with the child's eventual death.

During difficult discussions and queries it is necessary to use an unhurried approach, listen attentively, maintain good eye contact, paraphrase, and use reflective statements such as, "I know this is a difficult time for you and your son." Open body language is equally important and consists of sitting down at the same eye level and nodding and responding in a manner that ensures the nurse is attentive. Open-ended questions also enrich the discussions and convey a healing presence. Avoidance or poor eye contact often indicate discomfort with the conversation, anxiety, or disinterest. Family members and clients are very sensitive to nonverbal cues. Direct discussions and using eye contact while interacting with the client and family convey understanding and empathy.

Caring for seriously ill children and adolescents is replete with ethical dilemmas. Issues such as the child's participation in the decision-making process and communicating information regarding the youth's condition, medical prognosis, and treatment challenge nurses to develop ethically sound client-centered care that integrates the child and parent's psychosocial, cultural, and ethnic needs, values, and beliefs. Children's and adolescents' involvement in shared decision making is increasingly being advocated to ensure age-specific communication and emotional support during a stressful period. The nurse can encourage the child's participation through initiation of age-specific collaboration with the child and parents (Spence, 2000). Establishing partnerships with families strengthens their caregiving endeavors and the nurse–client relationship.

Prior to talking to seriously ill youths about death and dying issues it is very important for the nurse to have some knowledge of development issues concerning the child and family and their ability to communicate and comprehend the concept of death. According to Piaget's (1960) developmental theory, children lack a full comprehension of the finality of death until about 11 to 16 years of age. Despite this lack of full comprehension, researchers submit that children as young as 3 or 4 years old are able to acquire cues from physical changes in their bodies and nonverbal and verbal communication from nurses, staff, and their parents, resulting in advanced understanding of their disease and the concept of death (Sahler, Frager, Levetown, Cohn, & Lipson, 2000).

Age and developmental maturity determine how children grieve or cope with dying. Fears, uncertainty, and grief about death manifest differently in each child and adolescent, particularly in the latter stages of the illness; younger children often manifest their awareness and distress subtly. Fear of dying alone, being abandoned, and that death will be painful are widespread in children with chronic illnesses and end-of-life conditions (Stevens, 1998; Stevens, Jones, & O'Riordan, 1996). Sourkes (1992, 1996) describes the variations in coping styles of seriously ill children and adolescents in Table 3-1.

Experienced nurses can help students and novice nurses develop communication skills in this area by involving them in the care of a dying child. Situations involving a dying child provide opportunities to hear the questions youths raise about continuing treatment or stopping it altogether and to learn how to give compassionate and heartwarming responses. Communicating directly with the child who realizes he or she will die soon is one of the most rewarding ways to appreciate how the child really feels. Sahler and her colleagues (2000, p. 577) listed several questions dying children often raise, such as:

- "Can I have Pooh Bear with me?"
- "Will the doctors and nurses come to the funeral?"
- "Will Grandma be waiting for me in Heaven?"

Table 3-1 Common Coping Reactions in Seriously Ill Children and Adolescents

Age Group	Reactions
Younger children	A need to talk about death and dying
	Fears of losing parents
	Separation anxiety
	Sense of uncertainty
	Fear of abandonment
Older children	Fear of poor response to treatment
	Academic phobias
	Anxiety
	Regressive behaviors
Preadolescents	Anger
	Tearfulness
	Irritability
	Apathy
	Isolation
	Refusal to eat
	Uncooperativeness

Source: Sourkes, 1992; 1996.

Sahler et al. (2000) further submit that children often ask questions concerning the safeguarding of familiar and comforting people, places, and things that reassure them their lives have been meaningful and that they will not be forgotten. Dying alone is a common fear of dying children. Every measure should be used to ensure parents and other family members will be at the bedside when the child dies. Sometimes children ask questions about death and dying as a way to decide if it is safe or "okay" to discuss their fears and concerns with the nurse. Apart from verbal communication or expression of feelings, art and music therapy provide a creative venue for the child to express fears, anxiety, and distress. Throughout the child's treatment, the nurse must employ open and age-specific communication and relate to the youth and family in a respectful, empathetic manner and listen to and embrace what they say and believe.

Meghan is an 8-year-old who has a chronic history of cystic fibrosis. This is her third hospitalization within the past few months. During her morning care she asks the nurse questions about death and dying issues.

Meghan: Am I going to die?

Nurse: Tell me what you would like to know.

Meghan: Is it going to hurt?

Nurse: Is what going to hurt?

Meghan: Dying.

Nurse: We are going to make sure you are comfortable.

This nurse–client dialogue centered on reassuring the child that she will be comforted, supported, and not abandoned when she dies. This caring and compassionate response engenders trust and mitigates anxiety.

Working with seriously ill or dying children or adolescent is frequently very challenging to the nurse. Sensitive interactions surrounding the eminent death of a child often generates tremendous distress in the nurse and sometimes engenders "why does this child have to die" questions. It is essential for the nurse to acknowledge his or her feelings concerning these difficult situations to ensure objective and supportive care to seriously ill or dying children and their families. Only by getting to know the child and family can the nurse genuinely understand their experience and realize their unique needs (Luker, Austin, Caress, & Hallett, 2000; May, 1995).

Health education must be an integral part of communicating with and caring for youths and their families. Teaching parents the importance of engaging the child in age-specific activities (as tolerated), listening to their child's fears, giving the youth permission to die, fulfilling a child's wish (see Selected Web Sites: Make-A-Wish Foundation), and setting appropriate limits help the youth and parents cope with the child's eventual death (see Table 3-2). Closeness enriches the nurse–family relationship and creates a sense of connectedness and a therapeutic climate that fosters expression of feelings and discussion of personal wishes and expectations. Learning how to respond to the youth and family's fears and sense of hopelessness is essential during difficult situations. Open communication between the nurse and family, along with the family's and child's acknowledgment of the child's eventual death even while daily routines such as bathing, medication administration, and eating continue, move the family and child towards acceptance, provide quality-of-life experiences, and strengthen their ability to live in the present (Beale et al., 2005).

Embracing the youth's autonomy and independence and taking the youth's opinions, concerns, and treatment decisions seriously enhance communication among the nurse, youth, parents, and siblings. Although siblings have not been discussed extensively in this chapter, their needs along with other family members' concerns and fears must be assessed throughout treatment and addressed based on issues previously mentioned in this discussion.

Interactions involving the care of a dying or seriously ill child are fraught with intense emotions for both the child and the nurse. Death and dying raise questions about one's own mortality, and fear of dying sometimes raises questions about "why" a child has to die so young. Reviewing one's earliest experiences with death and sharing them with others is helpful in understanding one's present reactions to death. Self-awareness about death and dying issues is pivotal to nurses caring for dying clients, particularly young

Table 3-2 How to Communicate with the Terminally Ill Youth

1. Establish a time to talk to the youth while engaging in age-appropriate activities.
2. Listen to the child's fears, happiness, anger, or whatever the child wants to discuss.
3. Respect the child's wish not to talk about death.
4. Confirm the child's feelings without pressuring her or him to talk.
5. Engage in activities and conversations that foster a sense of autonomy and control.
6. Respect spiritual, ethnic, and cultural needs (e.g., prayers, saying grace with meals, etc).
7. Discuss the child and family's wishes regarding funding for community opportunities, such as the Make-A-Wish Foundation.
8. Reassure the child that he or she will not die alone and that he or she will be missed.

ones. The nurse must explore and embrace personal feelings; spiritual, cultural, and religious beliefs; past experiences with death; unresolved grief; and health care options associated with these issues. As the nurse becomes more secure with death and dying issues, the youth and parents are more likely to share their apprehension about these issues. Self-awareness bolsters the nurse's ability to attend to the client's emotional responses and manage stressful situations more proficiently.

A failure to recognize your feelings often impedes appreciation of the client's responses, inhibits their independence, and may result in "rescuing" or "avoiding" the client to cope with underlying personal reactions. Prolonged reactions such as tearfulness, crying, sadness, depression, irritability, recurrent thoughts of the dying client, and difficulty focusing or concentrating often signal unresolved grief issues associated with death and dying. Talking to a friend, colleague, religious advisor, or a spiritual support is helpful. If symptoms persist, talking to a trusted colleague or grief counselor or mental health professional is suggested. In essence, resolving feelings regarding end-of-life issues requires time, support, and education for the child, family, and nurse.

Middle Adulthood

The quality of care during the latter months of life has received growing attention during the past few years. Major findings show quality of life must be geared toward the client and his or her family's preferences, while actualizing optimal independence and self-efficacy. Integrating the client's wishes and needs into treatment planning is fundamental in devising client-centered health care that ensures quality end-of-life experiences and care. Families must be included in the decision-making process. They are an invaluable resource and provide information regarding their beliefs about the client's illness as well as the client's perspective of the end-of-life experience.

Most terminally or seriously ill clients, particularly middle-aged adults, want to know their diagnosis, participate in shared decision making, and be informed about their chances of survival. Uncertainties, worries, and fears engender a loss of control and sense of helplessness, resulting in a greater need for the nurse to collaborate with the health care team and share responsibility for decisions to implement client-centered health care. The nurse needs to advocate for client-centered care by strengthening the client's decision-making capacity through listening, addressing concerns, and health education. Effective nurse–client relationships correlate directly with the client's sense of control, competence, and satisfaction. Because of the interdisciplinary approach to care, the nurse must also be able to communicate with various team members and broker appropriate care and resources for the client and families coping with serious illnesses.

Middle-aged adults, like other age groups, benefit from specialized approaches that focus on treatment that integrates respect for the living and the dying. One model of end-of-life care recognized by the health and public sectors is hospice. **Hospice** is designed to provide comfort and support to clients and their families when a life-limiting illness no longer responds to cure-oriented treatments. Hospice care generally occurs in a home or community-based setting using an interdisciplinary approach. It enlists the family as a part of the client's care and values their perspectives and experiences as being just as important as the client's (Connor, Teno, Spence, & Smith, 2005; Teno, Clarridge, Casey, Edgman-Levitan, & Fowler, 2001).

Von Gunten and his colleagues (2000) developed a list of communication and relationship competencies to train physicians dealing with end-of-life situations. Although they were developed for physicians, they also are relevant to nurses working with adults facing end-of-life situations. The following are salient points from their seven-step approach for structuring communication concerning end of life:

- *Step 1: Prepare*—Nurses can gather accurate medical facts from interdisciplinary team discussions. Apart from clarifying the nature of the illness, an unhurried and accepting approach fosters an environment in which the nurse can appropriately assess the client's needs, wishes, preferences, values, beliefs, and culture.
- *Step 2: Clarify*—The nurse needs to clarify the client and family's knowledge of the client's condition, prognosis, and so on. Listening with interest is crucial to this process, as are open-ended questions and other communication skills that elicit knowledge concerning the client's condition. The nurse must anticipate an array of emotional responses. Because of the need to ensure privacy and confidentiality, the nurse must work with the interdisciplinary team to ensure consistent and accurate information is shared with the client and family.
- *Step 3: Ascertain how information will be communicated*—This particular step generates ethical and legal questions, particularly when the family opts to avoid telling the client about his true diagnosis and prognosis. This is a legal matter for the physician who must make a decision about the request based on client rights, wishes, values, and choices. However, this issue must be discussed in interdisciplinary team meetings to ensure everyone communicates the same message to the client and family members.

- *Step 4: Impart the information*—Again, health information or client education must be clear and consistent with the interdisciplinary team's recommendations. Consistent messages provide a sense of control and security and reduce anxiety and fears. Nurses must communicate the same information as other team members to ensure consistency and trust.
- *Step 5: Respond*—The nurse needs to respond appropriately to client and family emotions. Predictably, coping with end-of-life issues and decisions is very stressful and likely to generate an array of feelings, reactions, and emotions. Self-awareness of one's own perception of death is pivotal to this process. Open communication provides a supportive and safe environment of acceptance, empathy, and concern that enriches the nurse–client relationship.
- *Step 6: Develop a plan*—Develop a plan of care in which goals and treatment are prioritized and are negotiated among the client, family, and health care team. Negotiation of treatment goals and treatment priorities are discussed in depth. Agreement among the client, family, and health care team is likely to increase awareness of the client and health care team's expectation and open communication to clarify the client and family's needs, preferences, and health care practices.
- *Step 7: Devise a client-centered plan of care*—The client and family must be active participants in making health care decisions. This process requires open and honest communication among the client, family, and members of the interdisciplinary team concerning treatment options. Asking open-ended questions, imparting information, encouraging thoughts and feelings, and supporting client and family preferences, needs, health practices, unique circumstances, expectations, values, and beliefs all facilitate quality decision making. Overall, client needs are best met when principles of effective communication, ethical principles of self-determination, and the client's best interests are the cornerstone of client-centered decision making. (Von Gunten et al., 2000)

Predictably, during the treatment planning stage conflicts can arise between the nurse and other team members due to different perceptions and beliefs about death and dying issues, miscommunication, a lack of understanding or insight, or lack of attention by the family or provider. High tension and interpersonal conflicts between the client and/or family, the nurse, and other health professionals occur during this stage. The following nurse–client interaction is an example of a potential conflict situation involving a 68-year-old client suffering from end-stage chronic obstructive pulmonary disease (COPD) and her caregiver husband. This is the client's third hospitalization in the past 6 months. She has difficulty breathing despite treatment and is experiencing intense anxiety and fears of dying.

Spouse: I put the call light on 15 minutes ago and no one came. I know my wife is dying, but the nurses are ignoring her. That's not right!

Nurse: Mr. Jones, I understand you are pretty upset right now. I apologize for the delay in answering your wife's call light. How can I assist you?

Spouse: It is time for her "nerve" medication. Where is it?

Nurse: Let me check to see when she had her last dose and I'll be right back.

Spouse: I hope it doesn't take forever like it has in the past.

Nurse: I'll be right back.

Spouse: OK.

(The nurse returns in 3–5 minutes with antianxiety medication after she determines the client can have medication.)

Nurse: Mrs. Jones, I have your medication. Mr. Jones, I want to assure you that we want the best care for your wife. Please call me if you have further questions or concerns.

Spouse: I will. Everyone has really been OK. I apologize for losing my temper.

Nurse: I know this is a difficult time for you and your family, and believe me, Mrs. Jones, we plan to keep you as comfortable as possible. What else can I do for you?

This nurse–client interaction demonstrates the importance of remaining calm and displaying compassion, care, and concern. Remaining calm allowed the nurse to listen to and value the spouse's concerns and fears that generated anger, blaming, and a sense of powerlessness. Open-ended questions encourage expression of feelings and questioning, and ensures the information was understood. Through knowing the client and her spouse, and showing empathy and caring the nurse strengthened the nurse–client relationship and reaffirmed the best care for the client and the goal of collaborating to promote comfort and optimal quality of life. As already discussed, self-awareness regarding interpersonal conflicts is vital to facilitating effective nurse–client relationships.

CRITICAL THINKING QUESTION

You are doing a hospice home visit and the client's cousin asks, "How long is she expected to live?" She is persistent and asks you not to tell the client about her query.

Question: What is your best response?

A. Remind her that the client qualified for the hospice program because she is not expected to live.

B. Ask her if she has discussed this matter with the client and her family.

C. Acknowledge this must be a difficult time for the family, but remind her that health information is confidential.

Answer: Answer A is incorrect because it is evasive and lacks clarity. Answer B is also incorrect because it encourages her to ask the client about her condition. If the client and other family members wanted her to know they would have discussed it with her. Answer C is correct because obviously the cousin is concerned and this response conveys empathy. However, maintaining client confidentiality and privacy is an ethical and legal duty.

Older Adulthood

Older adulthood is a time of meaningful reflection and taking stock of one's life, relationships, integrity, quality of life, and sense of well-being. This is particularly challenging in societies that place tremendous emphasis on youth and have less respect for or a bias against aging. Looking back on one's life with a sense of fulfillment and wholeness, with positive regard, and as being full of integrity is considered mastery of the developmental issues inherent in aging. In contrast, a failure to feel whole and worthwhile and looking at life as unfulfilling or with discontent result in feelings of despair and that life was wasted. Older adults with a sense of integrity are more likely to cope with stressful life events than those with a sense of despair.

Debilitating or life-threatening illnesses and normal changes associated with aging place older adults at risk of employing ineffective coping responses, suffering, or dealing with complications associated with medical treatment.

As with other age groups, effective communication is necessary to establish healthy interpersonal relationships that ensure emotional support, as well as opportunities to express feelings and concerns. Older adults facing death experience similar emotional responses as other age groups, including feeling a loss of control, anger, denial, sadness, anxiety, and depression. Caring for older adults with end-of-life concerns requires an interdisciplinary approach to ensure holistic and client-centered treatment planning.

Respect for the client is pivotal in this process and requires embracing the aging process as a normal developmental stage, while avoiding stereotyping or making inappropriate assumptions about the client's decision-making abilities. Unless there is evidence of impaired cognitive function the client must be an active participant in the decision-making process. Ageism and other stereotypical assumptions about aging impede opportunities to collaborate with older adults. Some people are less distressed by end-of-life issues in older adults than in children or young people, perhaps because early death is viewed as unnatural and unfair. Exploring one's feelings about aging helps the nurse avoid stereotyping and distorting the client's experience. Although older adults are more hesitant to express their fears, thoughts, wishes, and preferences, nurses can strengthen the relationship through respect, acceptance, and support of these discussions. Each person views life and death differently, and the nurse must value and explore the individual's meaning of life, personal strengths, and support systems and value lifelong experiences and wisdom that contribute to how one copes with death and dying issues.

Communication with the older adult is sometimes difficult because of sensory deficits inherent in the aging process. Age-related sensory deficits such as hearing loss and visual disturbances are not synonymous with dementia or other cognitive disturbances that impair judgment and decision making; making such an assumption is stereotypical and biased. Effective communication begins with assessing the client's physical and psychosocial needs and unique concerns and wishes. Useful communication strategies for addressing age-related changes include the following:

• Use an unhurried approach.
• Speak to be heard and avoid shouting.
• Sit or stand directly in front of the client.
• Speak slowly and deliberately based on degree of sensory deficits.

- Use active listening skills.
- Remain nonjudgmental.
- Enlist family members.
- Assess the quality of his or her support system.
- Encourage storytelling to determine unique life experiences.
- Value the client's life experiences, wisdom, culture, beliefs, and preferences.

Applying these communication techniques conveys respect, sustains integrity, and creates a warm and safe environment in which the client trusts the nurse and feels safe and comfortable discussing fears, wishes, and wants about end-of-life concerns.

As with younger clients, older adults often fear dying alone, being abandoned, and being forgotten. Enlisting family members and friends mitigates some of the fears, anxiety, and uncertainties associated with dying. The nurse must extend every effort to respect and involve family members in the decision-making process. Explanations of diagnostic tests and procedures must be addressed in a respectful and sensitive manner to maintain family and older adult integrity and dignity.

Families play a key role in the care of clients facing death and dying issues. This is particular important when the client has cognitive deficits that impair memory and judgment needed to make end-of-life decisions pertaining to ethical and legal matters. Dying challenges the client and family to make critical decisions such as whether to limit or withhold life-sustaining treatment. Researchers submit that people approaching death often have a limited capacity to make these decisions. Clients have to cope with an array of symptoms that jeopardize their autonomy, including cognitive disturbances (e.g., delirium, dementia), severe pain, nausea, and extreme fatigue (Fann, 2000; Field & Cassel, 1997). Data further indicate about 30% of deaths occur in nursing homes, and a large percentage of these patients are debilitated and suffer from cognitive impairment (Fann). As mentioned earlier, the nurse must communicate with the client and family to ensure the client's wishes and rights are maintained even though he or she may be incapacitated. Even though the Patient Self-Determination Act and Cruzan decision by the Supreme Court imply that the client's choice concerning the protection of the client's interest at the end-of-life exists, Sullivan (2002) believes the decision falls short of explicating a process to implement these principles. Studies show that although most health professionals respect the client's freedom to make end-of-life decisions, freedom of choice is ambiguous and fails to guide care to preserve individual rights and decisions (Lynn et al., 2000; Molloy et al., 2000; Sullivan).

Issues involving the dying older adult, similar to other age groups, confront the nurse with complex ethical dilemmas that require nurse–client relationships that provide healing as well as supportive environments that facilitate open and honest discussions about end-of-life matters and feelings about the client's eventual death. Ethical and moral issues must also be communicated with staff and members of the interdisciplinary team. In a recent qualitative study (Oberle & Hughes, 2001), researchers compared physicians' and nurses' perceptions of ethical issues involving end-of-life decisions. Results from this study showed ethical decision making was difficult. Uncertainties about the optimal course of action for the client and family generated moral distress in this study. The fact that competing values reduce resources and that poor communication was common were also common themes of this study. Major difficulties for both physicians and nurses were based on witnessing suffering, which engendered a moral responsibility to reduce suffering. The researchers concluded that major differences between physicians and nurses were their roles in the decision-making process and moral motivation. Recommendations from these findings included the importance of physicians and nurses communicating with each other so they could understand and support the client, mitigate moral distress, and create strategies to resolve these issues (Oberle & Hughes).

Acknowledging and embracing the client's preferences for end-of-life care and their desire to communicate with the nurse, physician, and other members of the interdisciplinary treatment team ensure that the client's personal rights and dignity are maintained. As the broker of health care, nurses must establish interpersonal relationships with the client, family, and interdisciplinary team to implement the client's wishes. Poor or ineffective communication among the nurse, physician, and families often deprive the client of opportunities to share feelings about death and dying concerns. Interestingly, the physician and family members are generally unaware of the client's wishes and preferences due to physician uneasiness in discussing these issues, seeming time constraints, and diverse attitudes concerning the suitability of these discussions (Sahm, Will, & Hommel, 2005; Von Gunten et al., 2000). These barriers strengthen the argument that nurses must take the lead in advocating for timely dialogue among the client, family, and physician, though only if the client wishes to participate in these discussions. Specific communication approaches must respect culture, ethnicity, client and family preference, and beliefs about end-of-life matters. Paying close attention to the client and family members' communication needs may mitigate interpersonal conflict and reduce stress for all involved in the care of the dying client (see Chapter 4: Cultural Aspects of Communication Partnerships).

Equally important during this stressful period is the family caregiver's perspective and feelings about end-of-life decisions. In many cultures the family caregiver is the sole source of support for the client during the end-of-life period. The nurse must establish interactions with the family to ascertain the level of caregiver strain and how difficult it is for her or him to make decisions as to whether to withdraw or withhold life support for an aging loved one. Left unchecked, family caregiver strain and depression have deleterious effects on the caregiver's health and the client's functional level (Beach et al., 2005; Tilden, Tolle, Nelson, & Fields, 2001). Throughout the course of the client's illness the nurse must also assess the quality and availability of family caregivers' support systems. (See Research Study 3-2 on page 144.)

The following scenario demonstrates key concepts of end-of-life issues for families and nurses when confronted with ethical matters that generate strong emotions. It is important to respect decisions and offer support to resolve associated guilt, uncertainty, and despair.

Mrs. Jones is an 86-year-old client whose husband of 60 years is in the last stages of Alzheimer's disease. Although she is in for an annual checkup, she expresses despair because she can no longer care for him in their home, although she promised she would never put him in a nursing home. Her family urged her to put him in a nursing home 6 months ago, but she refused then because of her promise. She asks your opinion about putting the client in a nursing home.

Client: I feel very guilty about putting my husband in a nursing home. Do you think I made the right decision?

Nurse: I realize this is a difficult decision. Tell me what you know about your husband's condition.

Client: Well, he can no longer control his bodily functions and I am so tired and can't care for him at home anymore. The last time I came in the other nurse told me to keep him at home because I promised not to put him in a nursing home.

Nurse: I understand you have mixed feelings about putting your husband in the nursing home, but it sounds like you gave it a lot of thought and decided what was best for you. It sounds like the other nurse felt hopeful about your husband's condition.

Client: Well, do you think I made the right decision?

Nurse: As I said, I respect your right to do what you obviously think is best for you. I am sure your spouse knew you would make the best decision for your health and his. I can tell you were very close and loved each other.

Client: Thank you. I did do the best I could to keep my promise.

Nurse: By the way, how are you doing physically?

Client: I guess I'm okay; my doctor gave me a clean bill of health last year.

Nurse: Great. Sometimes taking care of a loved one makes it easy to forget about our own health. I just wanted to make sure you are taking care of yourself, too.

More and more nurses will be challenged by client and family decisions that generate strong personal feelings in the nurse. As previously discussed, self-awareness is critical to remaining objective and emotionally available to clients and families faced with making difficult decisions. The client's wife was torn between doing what she promised and taking care of herself and ensuring the client's safety. The nurse was able to convey empathy and understanding without allowing her feelings about the client's wife dilemma to effect her objective approach.

Clearly, effective and healthy nurse–client dialogue establishes trust and makes it easier for the client to express feelings and come to terms with emotionally intense decisions. Strengthening trust requires keeping promises; allowing clients to freely express their despair, and reiterating that emotional support and physical comfort are readily available (Buckman & Kason, 1992). Although the nature of life and death issues is painful, it is also necessary to provide emotional support and rely on interdisciplinary teams specializing in palliative or hospice care to process difficult situations. Quality interpersonal interactions with the client, family, and members of the health team are critical components of emotional support during difficult times. Nurses play key roles in developing client-centered health education and making appropriate community referrals unique to clients and families.

SUMMARY

In the face of rapid technological advances, there is a growing need to establish and employ collaborative relationships to ensure high-quality and effective communication among the nurse, clients, family, health care professionals, and other stakeholders. Effective communication skills are associated with positive health outcomes, greater shared decision making, appropriate goal setting, cost savings, higher client and staff satisfaction, and greater adherence to treatment. Recognition of the impact of nurse–client relationship amid dramatic societal and demographic changes and advances in telecommunication technologies continues to strengthen the need for the nurse to develop effective communication skills.

Nurse–client relationships must exist within a climate of warmth, caring, and empathy that ensures respect and dignity across the life span and health care continuum. Never before has there been a greater emphasis on communication skills and the nurse–client relationship. Technologies will never replace the face-to-face contact that facilitates rapport. This relationship serves several purposes including developing and maintaining a therapeutic relationship, data collection, shared decision making, support, health education, and collaborating and negotiating a plan of care. Nurses are at the forefront of the health arena and are the chief advocates of client-centered and holistic treatment across the continuum of care.

SUGGESTIONS FOR CLINICAL AND EXPERIENTIAL ACTIVITIES

1. Employ role-playing to practice how to establish trust and convey compassion in both an intense situation involving an angry client and a grave end-of-life situation.
2. Ask someone from a hospital's information technology (IT) department to educate you and your classmates about the importance of ensuring client privacy and confidentiality, and the strategies IT uses for this.
3. Invite a nurse ethicist or risk manager to discuss HIPAA guidelines and advance directives with the rest of your class.
4. Visit a medical center that has computerized medical records and demonstrate its efficiency in communicating important information among nurses and other health care professionals.
5. Break into small groups and discuss with your classmates your feelings about a dying child, adolescent, and older adult to assess personal feelings and improve self-awareness.
6. Use journaling to document personal reactions to end-of-life care.
7. Shadow an experienced palliative care nurse to learn about the impact of culture, ethnicity, and personal preferences on client questions, concerns, and fears.
8. Shadow a nurse providing hospice care and assess both the clients' and families' perceptions regarding end-of-life care.

END-OF-CHAPTER QUESTIONS

1. Peplau's Interpersonal Nursing Relations theory focuses on four stages of the nurse–client relationship. Which of the following demonstrates the Exploitation stage?
   a. The client is dependent on the nurse to lead communication and direct the client.
   b. The nurse and client use the collaborative process to establish holistic goal setting.
   c. The client expresses anger at the nurse and insists he needs to take charge of the conversations.
   d. The nurse has established trust and the client uses the relationship to advance health care needs.

2. The Internet and other telecommunication technologies enable the nurse and client to explore innovative communication processes. Of the following, which is accurate about telecommunications?
   a. The Internet and emails are equally effective in establishing nurse–client relationships.
   b. The Internet and emails are secure and cannot be accessed by others.
   c. Despite advances in information technologies, it is difficult to ensure client confidentiality and privacy.
   d. The Internet and email have not been proven to be efficient methods with which to communicate with the client.

3. Working with seriously ill children and their families challenges the nurse to explore personal reactions to end-of-life issues. Of the following, which indicates self-awareness?
   a. The nurse feels angry every time she takes care of the child.
   b. The nurse calls the parent to discuss the child, even when she is off duty.
   c. The nurse discusses her feelings with a trusted friend.
   d. The nurse has frequent interpersonal conflicts with the parents.

4. Nurses play key roles on the interdisciplinary team. Possessing assertive communication skills during meetings advances the needs of the client and family. Based on your understanding of collaboration, which best describes this concept?
   a. The nurse views him- or herself as a lone member who has to speak up for the client.
   b. The nurse views him- or herself as part of a team made up of various experts with similar goals.

      c. The nurse views him- or herself as a member of the team with less power than other members.

      d. The nurse views him- or herself as the leader of the team and makes the final decision about the client's care.

5. Mr. Jones is a 60-year-old man whose wife has been diagnosed with end-stage emphysema. During morning rounds he demands you take time to change the wife's linen and blames the hospital for mismanaging his wife's condition. Based on your understanding about family reactions to death or dying issues, what is the most appropriate response?

      a. Ignore him because he is obviously "having a bad day."

      b. Recognize that this may be his way of grieving and coping with feelings of helplessness.

      c. Ask him to stop yelling and get control of himself.

      d. Let him know how offended you are about his inappropriate behaviors.

Answers

5. b
4. b
3. c
2. c
1. d

Research Study 3–1

Title: Creating Opportunities for Parent Empowerment: Program Effects on the Mental Health/Coping Outcomes of Critically Ill Young Children and Their Parents. Melynk, B. M., Alpert-Gillis, L., Feinstein, N. F., Crean, H. F., Johnson, J., Fairbanks, E., et al. (2004). *Pediatrics, 113,* 597–607.

Study Problem/Purpose: The aim of the study was to evaluate the impact of a preventive educational-behavioral intervention, the Creating Opportunities for Parent Empowerment (COPE) program, initiated during early hospitalization on psychosocial outcomes for critically ill children and their parents.

Method: A randomized, controlled trial of 174 mothers and their 2- to 7-year-old children, with follow-up assessment 1, 3, 6, 9, and 12 months post hospitalization from pediatric ICU. Mothers in the COPE program participated in a 3-phase educational-behavioral intervention. The theoretical basis of the COPE program was self-regulation, control theory and emotional contagion theory.

Audiotapes and handouts as well as a parent-child work book were major teaching modalities.

Findings: Mothers who participated in the COPE program felt more confident, experienced less maternal stress regarding staff communication than control mothers, and had improved maternal and functional outcomes along with their children as compared to mothers who did not participate in this program.

Nursing Implications: Because hospitalization generates tremendous stress in both parents and children, nurses must assess their coping responses and establish shared-parent decision making and develop interventions that strengthen the parents coping skills in efforts to ameliorate negative consequences in their children.

Research Study 3–2

Title: Role Strain and Ease in Decision-Making to Withdraw or Withhold Life Support for Elderly Relatives. Hansen, L., Archbold, P. G., & Stewart, B. J. (2004). *Journal of Nursing Scholarship, 36, 233–238.*

Purpose: To identify and delineate concepts of role strain and role satisfaction (referred to as the ease in decision making) experienced by family caregivers when addressing decisions to withdraw or withhold life support for older adult relatives in diverse health care settings.

Method: Researchers used semistructured interviews and gathered data from 17 family caregivers to evaluate their experience when making end-of-life decisions about life support. Data from interviews were analyzed by content analysis.

Results/Findings: Analysis of the data revealed role strain was perplexing, interactive, and multifarious. The researchers concluded that their findings clarified the concept of role strain within the social context of life support decisions. Findings also indicate life support decision making by family members of older adults was not discreet and involved deliberations among family members.

Implications for Nursing: Because of the potential burden of decision making involving end-of-life decisions, the nurse must assess family caregivers' needs, experiences, and preferences to discuss this issue and intervene using collaborative relationships to facilitate dialogue.

REFERENCES

American Hospital Association Commission on Workforce for Hospitals and Health System. (2002). *In our hands: How hospital leaders can build a thriving workforce.* Chicago, IL: American Hospital Association.

Antai-Otong, D., & Wasserman, F. (2003). Therapeutic communication. In D. Antai-Otong (ed.), *Psychiatric Nursing: Biological and Behavioral Concepts* (pp. 127–150). Clifton Park, NY: Delmar Thomson Learning.

Baker, R., Mainous, A. G. III, Gray, D. P., & Love, M. M. (2003). Exploration of the relationships between continuity, trust in regular doctors and patient satisfaction with consultations with family doctors. *Scandinavian Journal of Primary Health Care, 21,* 27–32.

Balint, J., & Shelton, W. (1996). Regaining the initiative. Forging a new model of the patient-physician relationship. *Journal of the American Medical Association, 275,* 887–891.

Beach, S. R., Schulz, R., Williamson, G. M., Miller, L. S., Weiner, M. F., & Lance, C. E. (2005). Risk factors for potentially harmful informal caregiver behavior. *Journal of the American Geriatric Society, 53,* 255 –226.

Beale, E. A., Baile, W. F., & Aaron, J. (2005). Silence is not golden: Communicating with children dying from cancer. *Journal of Clinical Oncology, 23,* 3629–3631.

Blackhall, U., Murphy, S. T., Frank, G., Michel, V., Azen, S. (1995). Ethnicity and attitudes towards patient autonomy. *Journal of the American Medical Association, 274,* 820–825.

Bowers, B., Esmond, S., & Jacobson, N. (2000). The relationship between staffing and quality of long-term care facilities: Exploring the views of the nurse aides. *Journal of Nursing Care Quality, 14,* 55–64.

Buckman, R., & Kason, Y. (1992). *How to break bad news: A guide for health care professionals.* Baltimore, MD: John Hopkins University Press.

Chumbler, N. R., Mann, W. C., Wu, S., Schmid, A., & Kobb, R. (2004). The association of home-telehealth use and care coordination with improvement of function and cognitive functioning in frail elderly men. *Telemedicine Journal of e-Health, 10,* 129–137.

Collins, T. C., Clark, J. A., Petersen, L. A., & Kressin, N. R. (2002). Racial differences in how patients perceive physician communication regarding cardiac testing. *Medical Care, 40*(Suppl 1), 127–134.

Committee on Palliative and End-of-Life Care for Children and Their Families, Board on Health Sciences Policy, Institute of Medicine. (2003). *When children die: Improving palliative and end-of-life care for children and their families.* Washington, DC: National Academies Press.

Conger, K. J., Rueter, M. A., & Conger, R. D. (2000). The role of economic pressure in the lives of parents and their adolescents: The family stress model. In L. J. Crockett & R. J. Silbereisen (eds.), *Negotiating Adolescence in Times of Social Change* (pp. 201–233). Cambridge, England: Cambridge University Press.

Connor, S. R., Teno, J., Spence, C., & Smith, N. (2005). Family evaluation of hospice care: Results from voluntary submission of data via website. *Journal of Pain and Symptom Management, 30,* 9–17.

Davies, B., Steele, R., Collins, J. B., Cook, K., & Smith, S. (2004). The impact on families of respite care in a children's hospice program. *Journal of Palliative Care, 20,* 277–286.

Donadio, G. (2005). Improving healthcare delivery with the transformational whole person care model. *Holistic Nursing Practice, 19,* 74–77.

Elwyn, G., Edwards, A., Kinnersley, P., & Grol, R. (2000). Shared-decision making and the concept of equipoise: The competencies of involving patients in healthcare choices. *British Journal of General Practice, 50,* 892–899.

Eng, J. (2001). Computer network security for the radiology enterprise. *Radiology, 220,* 303–309.

Epstein, R. M. (1999). Mindful practice. *Journal of the American Medical Association, 282,* 833–839.

Eriksson, K. (2002). Caring science in a new key. *Nursing Science Quarterly, 15,* 61–65.

Etchells, F., Sharpe, G., Burgess, M. M., & Singer, P. A. (1996). Bioethics for clinicians: 2. Disclosure. *Canadian Medical Association, 155,* 387–391.

Eysenbach, G., & Diepgen, T. L. (1999). Patients looking for information on the Internet and seeking teleadvice: Motivation, expectations, and misconceptions as expressed in e-mails sent to physicians. *Archives of Dermatology, 135,* 151–156.

Eysenbach, G., & Jadad, A. R. (2001). Evidence-based patient choice and consumer health informatics in the Internet age. *Journal of Medical Internet Research, 3,* 319.

Fallowfield, L., Lipkin, M., & Hall, A. C. (1998). Teaching senior oncologists communication skills: Results from phase I of a comprehensive longitudinal program in the United Kingdom. *Journal of Clinical Oncology, 16,* 1961–1968.

Fann, J. R. (2000). The epidemiology of delirium: A review of studies and methodological issues. *Seminars in Clinical Neuropsychiatry, 5,* 2–12.

Faulkner, K. W. (1997). Talking about death with a dying child. *American Journal of Nursing, 97,* 64, 66, 68–69.

Feldman, P. H., Murtaugh, C. M., Pezzin, L. E., McDonald, M. V., & Peng, T. R. (2005). Just-in-time evidence-based email "reminders" in home healthcare: Impact on patient outcomes. *Health Service Research, 40,* 865–885.

Field, M., & Cassel, C. (1997). *Approaching death: Improving care at the end of life.* Washington, DC: Institute of Medicine, National Academy Press.

Fins, J. J., Miller, F. G., Acres, C. A., Bacchett, M. D., Huzzard, L. L., & Rapkin, B. D. (1999). End-of-life decision-making in the hospital: Current practice and future prospects. *Journal of Pain Symptom Management, 17,* 6–15.

Gill, J., & Mainous, A. L. (1998). The role of provider continuity in preventing hospitalizations. *Archives of Family Medicine, 7,* 352–357.

Gostin, L. O. (2001). Health information: reconciling personal privacy with the public good of human health. *Health Care Analysis, 9,* 321–335.

Grunfeld, E., Whelan, T. J., Zitzelsberger, L., Willan, A. R., Montesanto, B., & Evans, W. K. (2000). Cancer care workers in Ontario: Prevalence of burnout, job stress and job satisfaction. *Canadian Medical Association Journal, 163,* 166–169.

Halpern, J. (2001). *From detaches concern to empathy: Humanizing medical practice.* New York: Oxford University Press.

Hamann, J., Leucht, S., & Kissling, W. (2003). Shared decision making in psychiatry. *Acta Psychiatrica Scandinava, 107,* 401–402.

Hamvas, A., Wise, P. H., Yang, R. K., Wampler, N. S., Noguchi, A., et al. (1996). The influence of the wider use of surfactant therapy on neonatal mortality among blacks and whites. *New England Journal of Medicine, 334,* 1635–1640.

Harms, C., Young, J. R., Amsler, F., Zettler, C., Scheidegger, D., & Kindler, C. H. (2004). Improving anaesthetists' communication skills. *Anasthesia, 59,* 166–172.

Health Insurance Portability and Accountability Act of 1996. United States Public Law 104-191.

Heaven, C. M., & Maguire, P. (1997). Disclosure of concerns by hospice patients and their identification by nurses. *Palliative Medicine, 11,* 283–290.

Hilden, J. M., Emanuel, E. J., Fairclough, D. L., Link, M. P., Foley, K. M., Clarridge, B. C., et al. (2001). Attitudes and practices among pediatric oncologists regarding end-of-life care: Results of the 1998 American Society of Clinical Oncology Survey. *Journal of Clinical Oncology, 19,* 205–212.

Hinton, J. (1998). An assessment of open communication between people with terminal cancer, caring relatives, and others during home care. *Journal of Palliative Care, 14,* 15–23.

Horrigan, J. B., & Rainie, L. (2002). *Getting serious online.* Washington, DC: Pew Internet and American Life Project.

Institute of Medicine. (2001). *Crossing the quality chasm.* Washington, DC: National Academy Press.

Jarrett, N., & Payne, S. (1995). A selective review of the literature on nurse-patient communication: Has the patient's contribution been neglected? *Journal of Advanced Nursing, 22,* 72–78.

Jenkins, R., & Elliott P. (2004). Stressors, burnout, and social support: Nurses in acute mental health settings. *Journal of Advanced Nursing, 48,* 622–631.

Katz, R. L. (1963). *Empathy: Its nature and uses.* London, England: The Free Press of Glencoe.

Ketteridge, G., Delbridge, H., & Delbridge, L. (2005). How effective email communication for patients requiring elective surgery? *ANZ Journal of Surgery, 75,* 680–683.

Larson, D. G., & Tobin, D. R. (2000). End-of-life conversations: Evolving practice and theory. *Journal of the American Medical Association, 284,* 1573–1578.

Levinson, W., Roter, D. L., Mulloly, J. P., Dull, V. T., & Frankel, R. M. (1997). Physician-patient communication: The relationship with malpractice claims among primary care physicians and surgeons. *Journal of the American Medical Association, 277,* 553–557.

Liben, S. (1996). Pediatric palliative medicine: Obstacles to overcome. *Journal of Palliative Care, 12,* 24–28.

Lin, C. T., Wittevrongel, L., Moore, L., Beaty, B. L., & Ross, S. E. (2005). An Internet-based patient-provider communication system: Randomized controlled trial, 7, e47. Retrieved January 18, 2006, from http://www.jmir.org/2005/4/e47/

Lorig, K. R., Ritter P., Stewart, A. L., Sobel, D. S., Brown, B. W. Jr, Bandura, A., et al. (2001). Chronic disease self-management program: 2-year health status and health utilization outcomes. *Medical Care, 39,* 1217–1223.

Luker, K. A., Austin, L., Caress, A., & Hallett, C. E. (2000). The importance of "knowing the patient": Community nurses' constructions of quality in providing palliative care. *Journal of Advanced Nursing, 31,* 775–782.

Lynn, J., Devries, K. O., Arkes, H. R., Stevens, M., Cohn, F., Murphy, P., et al. (2000). Ineffectiveness of the SUPPORT intervention: A review of explanations. *Journal of the American Geriatrics Society, 48,* S206–S213.

Malasanos, T. H., Patel, B. D., Klein, J., & Burlingame, J. B. (2005). School nurse, family and provider connectivity in the FITE diabetes project. *Journal of Telemedicine and Telecare, 11*(Suppl 1), 76–78.

Mandl, K. D., Kohane, I. S., & Brandt, A. M. (1998). *Electronic patient-physician communication: Problems and promise. Annals of Internal Medicine, 129,* 495–500

Martin, M., Forchuk, C., Santopinto, M., & Butcher, H. (1992). Alternative approaches to nursing practice: Application of Peplau, Rogers, and Parse. *Nursing Science, 5,* 80–85.

Masera, G., Spinetta, J. J., Janovic, M., Ablin, A. R., D'Angio, G. J., Van Dongen-Melman, J., et al. (1999). Guidelines for assistance to terminally ill children with cancer: A report of the SIOP Working Committee on psychosocial issues in pediatric oncology. *Medical Pediatric Oncology, 32,* 44–48.

May, C. (1995). "To call it work somehow demeans it": The social construction of talk in the care of terminally ill patients. *Journal of Advanced Nursing, 22,* 556–561.

McCabe, C. (2004). Nurse-patient communication: An exploration of patients' experiences. *Journal of Clinical Nursing, 13,* 41–49.

McGilton, K. S., O'Brien-Pallas, L. L., Darlington, G., Evans, M., Wynn, F., et al. (2003). Effects of relationship-enhancing program of care on outcomes. *Image: Journal of Nursing Scholarship, 35,* 151–156.

Meier, D. E., Back, A. L., & Morrison, R. S. (2001). The inner life of physicians and care of the seriously ill. *Journal of the American Medical Association, 286,* 3007–3017.

Melnyk, B. M., Alpert-Gillis, L., Feinstein, N. F., Crean, H. F., Johnson, J., Fairbanks, E., et al. (2004). Creating opportunities for parent empowerment: Program effects on the mental health/coping outcomes of critically ill young children and their mothers. *Pediatrics, 113,* 597–607.

Melnyk, B. M., Alpert-Gillis, L. J., Hensel, P. B., Cable-Billing, R. C., & Rubenstein, J. S. (1997). Helping mothers cope with a critically ill child: A pilot test of the COPE intervention. *Research Nursing Health, 20,* 3–14.

Messmer, P. R., Rodriquez, S., Adams, J., Wells-Gentry, J., Washburn, I., Zabaleta, I., et al. (1997). Practice applications of research. Effect of kangaroo care on sleep time in neonates. *Pediatric Nursing, 23,* 408–414.

Molloy, D. W., Guyatt, G. H., Russo, R., Goeree, R., O'Brien, B. J., Bedard, M., et al. (2000). Systematic implementation of an advance directive program in nursing homes: A randomized, controlled trial. *Journal of the American Medical Association, 283,* 1437–1444.

Morrison, R. S., Chichin, E., Carter, J., Burack, O., Lantz, M., & Meier, D. E. (2005). The effect of a social work intervention to enhance advance care planning documentation in the nursing home. *Journal of the American Geriatrics Society, 53,* 290–294.

Morse, J. (1991). Negotiating commitment and involvement in the nurse-client relationships. *Journal of Advanced Nursing, 16,* 455–468.

Nauhauser, L., & Kreps, G. L. (2003). Rethinking communication in the e-health era. *Journal of Health Psychology, 8,* 7–23.

Novack, D. H., Suchman, A. L., Clark, W., Epstein, R. M., Najberg, E., & Kaplan, C. (1997). Calibrating the physician: Personal awareness and effective patient care. *Journal of the American Medical Association, 278,* 502–509.

Oberle, K., & Hughes, D. (2001). Doctors' and nurses' perception of ethical problems in end-of-life decisions. *Journal of Advanced Nursing, 33,* 707–715.

Patient Self-Determination Act of 1990. Pub. L. No. 101-508, ss 4206, 104 Stat. 1388.

Peplau, H. E. (1952). *Interpersonal relations in nursing.* New York: G. P. Putnam.

Peplau, H. E. (1991). *Interpersonal relations in nursing: A conceptual frame of reference for psychodynamic nursing.* New York: Springer.

Phillips, R. B., & Moses, H. A. (1996). Skin hunger effects on preterm neonates. *Infant Toddler Intervention: The Transdisciplinary Journal, 6,* 39–46.

Piaget, J. (1960). *The child's conception of the world.* Paterson, NJ: Littlefield.

Purcell, G. P., Wilson, P., & Delamothe, T. (2002). The quality of health information on the Internet. *British Medical Journal, 324,* 557–558.

Rafiq, A., & Merrell, R. C. (2005). Telemedicine for access to quality care on medical practice and continuing medical education in a global arena. *Journal of Continuing Education in the Health Professions, 25,* 34–42.

Richardson, J. (2002). Health promotion in palliative care: The patient's perception of therapeutic interaction with the palliative nurse in the primary care setting. *Journal of Advanced Nursing, 40,* 432–440.

Riva, G. (2002). The sociocognitive psychology of computer-mediated communication: The present and future of technology-based interactions. *Cyberpsychology Behavior, 5,* 581–598.

Roden, J. (2005). The involvement of parents and nurses in the care of acutely-ill children in a non-specialist paediatric setting. *Journal of Child Health Care, 9,* 222–240.

Roter, D. L., Stewart, M., Putnam, S. M., Lipkin, M. Jr, Stiles, W., & Inui, T. S. (1997). Communication patterns of primary care physicians. *Journal of the American Medical Association, 277*, 350–356.

Roy, C. (1970). Adaptation: A conceptual framework for nursing. *Nursing Outlook, 18*, 42– 45.

Roy, C. (1984). *Introduction to nursing: An adaptation model* (2nd ed.). Englewood Cliffs, NJ: Prentice-Hall.

Roy, C., & Andrews, H. A. (1999). *The Roy adaptation model* (2nd ed.). Stamford, CT: Appleton & Lange.

Rundqvist, E. M., & Severinssion E. I. (1999). Caring relationships with patients suffering from dementia—an interview study. *Journal of Advanced Nursing, 29*, 800–807.

Sahler, O. J., Frager, G., Levetown, M., Cohn, F. G., & Lipson, M. A. (2000). Medical education about the end-of-life care in the pediatric setting: Principles, challenges, and opportunities. *Pediatrics, 105*, 575–584.

Sahm, S., Will, R., & Hommel, G. (2005). Attitudes towards and barriers to writing advance directives among cancer patients, healthy controls, and medical staff. *Journal of Medical Ethics, 31*, 437–440.

Silberg, W. M., Lundberg, G. D., & Musacchio, R. A. (1997). Assessing, controlling, and assuring the quality of medical information on the Internet. *Journal of the American Medical Association, 277*, 1244–1245.

Siminoff, L. A., & Step, M. M. (2005). A communication model of shared decision making: Accounting for cancer treatment decisions. *Health Psychology, 24*(Suppl 4), S99–S105.

Sourkes, B. M. (1992). The child with a life-threatening illness. In J. Brandell (ed.), *Countertransference in Psychotherapy with Children and* Adolescents (pp. 267–284). New York: Jason Aronson.

Sourkes, B. M. (1996). The broken heart: Anticipatory grief in the child facing death. *Journal of Palliative Care, 12*, 56–59.

Spence, G. E. (2000). Children's competency to consent: An ethical dilemma. *Journal of Children's Health Care, 4*, 117–122.

Spielberg, A. R. (1999). Online without a net: Physician-patient communication by electronic mail. *American Journal of Law Medicine, 25*, 267–295.

Stephan, W. G., & Finlay, K. A. (1999). The role of empathy in improving intergroup relations. *Journal of Social Issues, 55*, 729–743.

Stevens, M. M. (1998). Psychological adaptation of the dying child. In D. Doyle, G. W. C. Hanks, & N. MacDonald (Eds.), *Oxford Textbook of Palliative Medicine* (2nd ed., pp. 1057–1075). New York: Oxford University Press.

Stevens, M. M., Jones, P., & O'Riordan, E. (1996). Family responses when a child with cancer is in palliative care. *Journal of Palliative Care, 12*, 51–55.

Stewart, M., Brown, J. B., Boon, H., Galajda, J., Meredith, L., & Sangster, M. (1999). Evidence on patient-doctor communication. *Cancer Prevention and Control, 3*, 25–30.

Stewart, M. A. (1996). Effective physician-patient communication and health outcomes: A review. *Canadian Medical Association Journal, 152,* 1423–1433.

Sullivan, M. D. (2002). The illusion of patient choice in end-of-life choices. *American Journal of Geriatric Psychiatry, 10,* 365–372.

Sullivan, M. (2003). The new subjective medicine: Taking the patient's point of view on health care and health. *Social Science Medicine, 56,* 1595–1604.

Taylor, H. (May 1, 2002). *Cyberchondriacs update.* Harris Poll No. 21. Retrieved August 8, 2005, from http://www.harrisinteractive.com

Teno, J. M., Clarridge, B., Casey, V., Edgman-Levitan, S., & Fowler, J. (2001). Validation of a toolkit after death—bereaved family member interview. *Journal of Pain and Symptom Management, 22,* 752–758.

Teno, J. M., Fisher, E., Hamel, M. B., Wu, A. W., Murphy, D. J., Wenger, N. S., et al. (2000). Decision-making and outcomes of prolonged ICU stays in seriously ill patients. *Journal of the American Geriatric Society, 48*(Suppl 5), S70–S74.

Tilden, V. P., Tolle, S. W., Nelson, C. A., & Fields, J. (2001). Family decision-making to withdraw life-sustaining treatment from hospitalized patients. *Nursing Research, 50,* 105–115.

Tobin, D. R. (1999). *Peaceful dying.* Reading, MA: Perseus.

Tulsky, J. A. (2005). Beyond advance directives. Importance of communication skills at the end of life. *Journal of the American Medical Association, 294,* 359–365.

Von Gunten, G. F., Ferris, F. D., & Emanual, L. L. (2000). Ensuring competency in end-of-life care: Communication and relational skills. *Journal of the American Medical Association, 284,* 3051–3057.

Wanzer, M. B., Booth-Butterfield, M., & Gruber, K. (2004). Perceptions of health care providers' communication: Relationships between patient-centered communication and satisfaction. *Health Communication, 16,* 363–383.

Whalen v. United States, 429 United States 58, 1966.

Wolfe, J., Friebert, S., & Hilden, J. (2002). Caring for children with advanced cancer: Integrating palliative care. *Pediatric Clinics of North America, 49,* 1043–1062.

SELECTED WEB SITES

Alzheimer's Association: http://www.alz.org

Alzheimer's Association Diversity Toolbox:
http://www.alz.org/Resources/Diversity/overview.asp

American Academy of Pediatrics: www.pediatrics.org

Health Insurance Portability and Accountability Act of 1996 (HIPAA):
http://www.cms.hhs.gov/HIPAAGenInfo/

Hospice Association of America: http://www.hospice-america.org

Hospice Foundation of America: http://www.hospicefoundation.org

Institute of Medicine—Reading materials about technology and health-related problems: http://www.iom.edu

Make-A-Wish Foundation—Charitable organization that grants wishes to children with life-threatening medication conditions: http://www.wish.org

The National Hospice and Palliative Care Organization—Information available in English and Spanish: http://www.nhpco.org

PBS Children's Hospital Parents Center: http://www.pbs.org/opb/childrenshospital/parents

Decision Support Tools

Agency for Healthcare Research and Quality: http://www.ahrq.gov

Cochrane Collaboration: http://www.cochrane.org

DynaMed: http://www.dynamicmedical.com

Improving Chronic Illness Care (ICIC): http://www.improvingchroniccare.org

Medscape/WebMD: http://www.webmd.com

National Guideline Clearinghouse: http://www.guideline.gov

Chapter Four

Cultural Aspects of Communication Partnerships

LEARNING OBJECTIVES

Upon completion of this chapter, the reader should be able to:

1. Define culture and its impact on nurse–client relationships

2. Describe major components of cultural competence

3. Discuss the significance of self-awareness on how one interprets the experiences and health care and emotional needs of others

4. Delineate major concepts of Leininger's transcultural nursing theory

5. Analyze the role of culture in nurse–client relationships across the life span

KEY TERMS

Beliefs—A set of convictions that have meaning to the individual, group, family, or community.

Cultural competence—A set of knowledge, skills, behaviors, and policies that help clinicians to form therapeutic relationships, convey empathy and sensitivity, and collaborate and work effectively with diverse populations.

Cultural space—The unique meaning of physical and interpersonal distance within a sociocultural context.

Culture—The totality of learned and transmitted behaviors, beliefs, and values shared within a social context, including language, communication patterns, customs, rituals, and health practices.

Ethnicity—A group sharing a common and distinctive culture, allegiance, religion, or language.

Linguistic competence—The capacity to converse or to communicate information in a manner readily understood by diverse populations, including those with limited English proficiency.

Linguistics—Pertains to the systematic study or understanding of language and includes phonetics, patterns of nonverbal and verbal gestures, semantics, and pragmatics. Human language is a natural phenomenon and language learning is common in childhood within sociocultural contexts.

Values—A set of principles or standards unique to a culture and/or ethnicity; a measure of qualities that determine usefulness and significance to the individual.

INTRODUCTION

"One of the greatest challenges in nursing is to discover how culture care factors can make a difference in understanding others and providing meaningful and satisfying nursing care to those served" (Leininger, 1995, p. 115). The seminal contributions of Madeleine Leininger, founder and principal leader of transcultural care, are vast. Her research and numerous publications involving human caring within a cultural context continue to shape client-centered and holistic nursing care (Leininger, 1996, 2002). Transcultural care focuses on a holistic or client-centered approach that facilitates congruent and meaningful care. Respecting the client's individuality is the basis of nursing.

Culture frames the way in which people perceive the world and impacts interactions within social contexts. Broadly defined, **culture** refers to a way of life of a group or person (Stewart, 1995). It shapes the totality of learned and transmitted behaviors, customs, mores, and values shared within a social context (Leininger, 1991), which includes language, gender, generation, communication patterns, customs, and health practices. **Cultural competence** is a compilation of knowledge, skills, behaviors, and policies that help clinicians to collaborate and work effectively with diverse populations. Campinha-Bacote (1999) defines cultural competence as "the process in which the healthcare worker strives to achieve the ability to work within the cultural context of a client (individual, family, or community)" (p. 203). Based on this definition, cultural competence can be seen as a developmental process that evolves over time (Campinha-Bacote, 1995; Cross, Bazron, Dennis, & Isaacs, 1989; Leininger, 1995; Leininger & McFarland, 2006; Purnell, 2000). Cultural competence occurs when the nurse translates and integrates knowledge of the client's uniqueness, wishes, and preference into the nurse-client relationship and client-centered care planning. Client-centered approaches facilitate positive nurse–client relationships, involve the client in shared decision making, and advance quality clinical care.

Each client brings a rich diversity of experiences, values, wishes, preferences, religious beliefs, linguistic backgrounds, and health practices to the domains in which illness and health occur. Several issues that guide the client's language and perception of self and others include values, beliefs, and linguistics. **Values** pertain to the worth or significance that determines merit, usefulness, or significance. **Beliefs** refer to mental acceptance of the truth or actuality of something. Something accepted as the truth. **Linguistics** refer to the study and understanding of language within a specific social context. Collectively, these aspects of the client are the basis of culturally sensitive and competent nursing care. It is noteworthy to mention that although cultural differences shape the client's understanding of the meaning of life experiences, health practices, beliefs, and values, some commonalities exist across all cultures, such as the right to equitable access to health care, respect from others and the provision of safety for children and other vulnerable populations (Leininger, 1985).

Cultural distinctions between the nurse and client are also clinically significant (Lockhart & Resnick, 1997). Culture is the basis of the client's experiences, so nurses must expand their knowledge base and discover how various cultures contribute to holistic and client-centered care. Discovering these perspectives and the potential impact of one's own culture on the client's perspective is crucial to the nurse–client interaction. Personal traditions and culture influence nurse–client interactions both consciously and unconsciously. The nurse perceives the client's experiences through the subjective lens of his or her own personal culture, customary beliefs, and values. Additional factors that influence cultural beliefs and customs include religion and spirituality. Religious and spiritual experiences are among the most important cultural factors shaping beliefs, values, mores, and perceptions of health and illness (Krippner & Welch, 1992). Religious and spiritual beliefs are often an integral part of the client's culture and determine how one dresses, expresses thoughts and emotions, interacts with elders, and determines the role and responsibilities of men, women, children, and older adults. A failure to consider these factors may have an adverse impact on the nurse–client relationship and communication with family members. As each client is seen as an individual who practices within a specific sociocultural context, the nurse is better prepared to identify issues unique to the client and collaborate with him or her more effectively and develop and implement client-centered health care. Client-centered health care is every person's right. When nurses treat patients with respect and dignity, listen to their concerns, impart information, and maintain open communication, therapeutic relationships are strengthened and client satisfaction is enhanced.

Respecting the client's individuality and implementing holistic care through nurse–client relationships requires a comprehensive, culturally based assessment that incorporates the client's and family's wishes and preferences and involves them in participatory decision making. This approach facilitates individualized health care. Moreover, how the nurse explains or interprets the client's complaints and perceptions of health and illness must be guided by knowledge of individual client needs rather than by the nurse's subjective opinion. Imposing personal values and beliefs on the client jeopardizes trust, dignity, and respect, all of which are critical to effective communication among the nurse, client, and family. Ultimately, cultural insensitivity results in poor interpersonal relationships, frustration in the nurse and client, mistrust, health care disparities, and poor health outcomes. The nurse who establishes rapport and trust and maintains a quality interpersonal relationship with the client and family conveys empathy, respect, and value of differences. The role of effective interpersonal care in optimizing clinical outcomes must not be underestimated. Through healthy nurse–client interactions, the client believes the nurse accepts his or her culture, ethnicity, age, language, gender, health practices, and customs. **Ethnicity** refers to unique characteristics, such as race, common traits, customs, language, social views or affiliation of the individual, family, community, or society. Because of the importance of quality nurse–client relationships and shared decision making, nurses must transcend these differences through self-awareness and a willingness and capacity to become culturally competent and sensitive.

Students as well as novice and experienced nurses must be prepared to respond to and assess the needs of diverse cultural groups and develop mutual goals and treatment plans to ensure client satisfaction, symptom relief, adherence to treatment, and positive clinical outcomes. Cultural discord frequently exists when the client's subjective experiences of health-related problems, preferences, and health practices differ from the nurse's approach to health care problems (Helman, 1990). Understanding and respecting cultural beliefs and involving the client in shared decision making facilitates quality nursing care.

Although culture is discussed throughout this book, this chapter focuses primarily on communication within the social context of culture, ethnicity, and individuality of clients of all ages seeking health care. It also provides an overview of major transcultural theories and implications for nursing practice. While this chapter focuses primarily on the cultural components of communication directed by changing demographics and disparities in health care, each client must be respected for his or her uniqueness.

CHANGING DEMOGRAPHICS

In 2000, the U.S. Census Bureau (Hobbs & Stoops, 2002) stated that more than 30% of the U.S. population could be considered an ethnic minority (anything other than non-Hispanic white). More than 50% of the population is expected to be in this group by 2050 (U.S. Census Bureau, 2000). As societies become more pluralistic, nurses will have daily encounters with clients of various cultures, ethnicities, and socioeconomic backgrounds. Two major issues facing nursing are the high percentage of non-Hispanic white nurses caring for this growing minority and the underrepresentation of registered nurses from diverse cultures and ethnicities (American Association of Colleges of Nurses [AACN], 2001; Gardner, 2005; Trossman, 1998; U.S. Department of Health and Human Services, 2001).

An even more challenging issue confronting today's nurse is an enormous need to provide quality and culturally sensitive health care to a pluralistic society with diverse health care needs. This challenge begins with nursing students and nurse educators and includes all nurses. The underrepresentation of nurses from diverse cultural and ethnic backgrounds complicates this picture, making it imperative for all nurses to seek avenues to prepare for an increasingly pluralistic society. A growing concern among nurse educators and minority nursing students is the necessity to prepare all students to care for individuals from varied backgrounds. This process must begin with nurse educators who set the tone, define expectations, and provide role models for students to become cognizant of their own culture, ethnicity, mores, motivation, and values and how they shape sensitivity and perceptions of others. Gardner (2005) states that the efforts of nurse educators must extend beyond "agreeing that culture diversity should be a goal of higher education" (p. 161) and submits that there is a critical need for educators to communicate empathy and caring to nursing students to reduce the high attrition rate among minority students. Empathy includes open communication, a willingness to listen, showing understanding of personal stressors, and providing emotional support. In addition, Gardner emphasized the need for educators to become more knowledgeable of or culturally sensitive to the needs of students from diverse backgrounds and ethnicities. A culturally diverse nursing profession is critical to the integrity of nursing and its ability to address the unique health needs of individuals across the life span (AACN, 2001). A growing number of colleges and universities have developed innovative recruitment programs to attract diverse populations. Education must extend beyond nurse educators to include students, and must focus on culture, communication, implicit bias, and self-awareness (Gardner; Hilgenberg & Schlickau, 2002). (See Research Study 4-1 on page 187 for a discussion of Gardner's qualitative study of minority nursing students' experiences.)

Working with diverse cultures and ethnicities requires cultural competence and sensitivity. Students, novices, and experienced nurses can strengthen cultural competence through innovative strategies, such as using case studies of diverse populations as an Internet collaborative learning activity aimed at improving transcultural knowledge (Byers, Hilgenberg, & Rhodes, 1999; Hilgenberg & Schlickau, 2002). Hilgenberg and Schlickau developed such an activity, based on Leininger's (1991) Sunrise Model (discussed more fully later in this chapter). The two case studies involved a Mexican American family and an Amish family and were available in hard copy and on each faculty member's Web page. Major goals of the students' assignments included:

• Formulate a comprehensive knowledge concerning a specific cultural group.
• Problem solve with peers to formulate a culturally congruent plan of care to meet the holistic client needs of families described in the case studies.
• Apply Leininger's theory to the Amish and Hispanic cultures.
• Compare similarities and differences between the two cultures.
• Identify health-related situations from each cultural perspective.

Results of this activity revealed that using the Internet for peer collaboration and retrieval of dialogue enhanced the students' computer literacy and knowledge, as well as improving their skills in transcultural nursing (Hilgenberg & Schlickau, 2002).

Faculty, students, and nurses must seek opportunities such as this one to enhance culturally competent care. As nursing faculty pave the way and open communication channels that stimulate dialogue and problem solving with diverse groups, students will take notice and recognize how their own culture can be an asset or a liability in creating healthy encounters with all clients.

Because culture shapes attitudes, behaviors, health practice, values, and beliefs, nurses face growing pressure to form quality nurse–client relationships and communicate with and care for individuals from diverse populations. A significant aspect of establishing these relationships is a willingness to understand the client's experiences. Western society explains health and illness using scientific reasoning, whereas diverse cultures explain illness and health as being mystical or emotional; as being based on superstition, charms, ghosts, or religious or spiritual beliefs; as being a punishment, or caused by evil or "spells"; or as being an imbalance of hot and cold sensations or of yin and yang (Giger & Davidhizar, 2004; Leininger & McFarland, 2006; Padilla, Gomez, Biggerstaff, & Mehler, 2001; Vivian & Dundes, 2004). Evaluating the role of healers and religious leaders in various cultures affords a glimpse of health practices and beliefs and their impact on the client's perception of illness and health. Matters are complicated when the client's explanation of symptoms and the nurse's explanation of symptoms clash or differ. A lack of knowledge and an unwillingness to communicate with the client or involve him or her in care planning is likely to compromise the nurse–client relationship and result in misdiagnosis, inappropriate goal setting, and negative clinical outcomes. Given the tremendous increase in the variety of cultures in the United States, nurses and other clinicians are increasingly likely to encounter individuals from diverse groups across the health care continuum. A failure to assess the client's needs and experience from a sociocultural perspective widens the gap between the nurse and client and compromises the implementation of appropriate and quality health care.

HEALTH CARE DISPARITIES

A growing concern among health care leaders and some lawmakers is the racial and ethnic disparities in health care access and quality (Mayberry, Mili,

& Ofili, 2000). Healthy People 2010 defines health disparities as distinctions in disease prevalence or access to treatment based on gender, race, ethnicity, socioeconomic status, sexual orientation, geographic locale, or education (U.S. Department of Health and Human Services, 2000). Although there is no consensus concerning the sole cause of disparities in health care, some researchers have identified contributing factors and potential barriers. Contributing factors associated with health disparities include client preferences, poor communication with clinicians, alienation, mistrust, and access difficulties. From a broader perspective, disparities in health care are linked to historic and modern social and economic disparities, bias, stereotyping, prejudice, and a lack of cultural sensitivity or competence among nurses and other clinicians, especially physicians (Carrasquillo, Orav, Brennan, & Burstin, 1999; Cooper-Patrick et al., 1999; Malat, 2001). Causes of health care disparities extend beyond the nurse and other clinicians and include the culture of the health care system.

Racial, ethnic, and linguistic biases have existed for more than three centuries (Byrd & Clayton, 2000, 2002; Gamble, 1997). Emerging evidence indicates these variables contribute to poor access to care, bias and stereotyping, and a failure to communicate and understand the meaning of the client's experience; they also are related to poor clinical outcomes, alienation, and mistrust toward health care providers and health care systems. Although awareness of health disparities has increased over the past 20 years or so, they persist, particularly regarding women, various age groups (Epstein, 1999; Jerant, Franks, Jackson, & Doescher, 2004; Murphy, Krumholz, & Gross, 2004), and minority groups, no matter the client's level of insurance, income, or education (Persell & Baker, 2004; Schulman et al., 1999; Smedley, Stith, & Nelson, 2003).

Demographic changes forecast for the next decade expand the significance of addressing and reducing racial and ethnic disparities in health care and ensuring equitable health care to all citizens. Although significant efforts to improve access to quality health care and to reduce health disparities have occurred the past few years, these problems still exist among minorities, women, older adults, and poorly educated populations (Mullins, Blatt, Gbarayor, Yang, & Baquet, 2005). Strategies to eliminate disparities must concentrate on cultural sensitivity or competence among nurses and other clinicians to improve health care access and health education.

Effective communication among the nurse, client, and family requires a purposeful approach to shore up cultural competence and sensitivity to all clients. Although reducing health disparities is a major focus of cultural competence, a basic approach of understanding and appreciating the uniqueness of all clients begins the process. Cultural sensitivity and cultural competence can be facilitated by:

- Employing effective communication through active listening
- When appropriate, using interpreters to manage language barriers in individuals with limited English proficiency
- Conveying respect for and the value of tribal relationships
- Using factual understanding of the client's experience

Communication difficulties due to cultural differences between the nurse and the client/family frequently dilute the client's knowledge about his or her illness and the health and treatment options available. Communication or linguistic differences also reduce nurse–client connectedness. The nurse must pursue and implement strategies that foster effective communication to accurately interpret client complaints, promote comfort, and provide venues for the client to express feelings and concerns. Nurses, like other clinicians, have a moral and ethical obligation to use effective communication skills to assess and seek knowledge concerning cultural and individual needs. Although the primary focus of this chapter is cultural competence as a necessary communication skill, some nurse leaders contend that cultural competence *is* nursing competence (Dreher & Macnaughton, 2002). Nursing competence transcends culture, race, gender, age, and ethnicity and requires the provision of holistic interventions to advance quality clinical outcomes. It is also a lifelong process involving a willingness to seek to know and understand others from an objective and factual perspective.

Núñez (2000) contends that most encounters involve a tricultural interaction among the nurse, the client, and the health care system. Together, these factors shape the nurse–client encounter, the client's involvement in treatment planning, and his or her response to health care. For example, a nurse could have a strong Pennsylvania Dutch cultural background, the client could be a naturalized South African, and the health care system is in rural Utah. In this situation cultural competence is most likely to occur when the nurse recognizes the potential effect of her or his own culture on how she or he communicates, understands, assesses, and translates the meaning of the client's experiences and responsiveness to health care needs. Self-awareness is a core feature of cultural sensitivity and individualized care. It is imperative to learn how one's culture influences the interpretation of the experiences of clients from different cultures and the client's behavior toward the nurse. Through this lens of self-awareness, the nurse acquires a global understanding of transactions among various cultures instead of stereotyping the characteristics of diverse groups (Núñez). The success of self-awareness depends on the nurse's willingness and motivation to address personal values, feelings, and behaviors that direct understanding and knowledge of diverse populations.

Quality of care is related to accessibility and equitable health care. Hence, it is logical to assume that eliminating health care disparities is every health clinician's responsibility. Nurses and other clinicians must develop and implement individualized approaches that enhance communication and ultimately reduce health disparities and increase equitable and timely access to care. Cultural competence requires knowledge of theories that guide the nurse in identifying and understanding the diversity each client brings to each encounter and how personal culture governs this process. The following communication considerations of cultural competence provide a basis and guide for discovering the distinctiveness of each client and for internalizing the motivation and capacity to become culturally sensitive and expand holistic health care.

COMMUNICATION CONSIDERATIONS OF CULTURAL COMPETENCE

Knowing the significance of nurse–client holistic care across the health continuum, efforts to understand client experiences, improve communication, and foster trust among diverse cultures and ethnicities must be a priority. Open, nonjudgmental, and honest communication offers the nurse a way in which to interact with diverse cultures to identify and evaluate their needs and preferences. Predictably, effective communication between the nurse and client is more difficult when there are cultural and linguistic barriers. Health care systems must address **linguistic competence** to ensure accurate and appropriate communication of information in languages other than English. **Linguistic competence** refers to the nurse's ability to understand language, both verbal and nonverbal cues and symbols unique to the individual, family and community. Nurse–client encounters provide forums to understand the meaning of the client's experiences, concerns, preferences, and health practices through cross-cultural communication. Compelling evidence demonstrates that positive clinical outcomes, client satisfaction, and adherence to treatment may be a result of cross-cultural communication in which the client's needs, preferences, and wishes are respected and integrated into treatment (Cooper-Patrick et al., 1999; Institute of Medicine [IOM], 2001; Laine & Davidoff, 1996; Stewart et al., 1999). Unresolved language barriers result in poor access to preventive services, higher rates of chronic disease, poor disease management, and negative clinical outcomes (Lieu et al., 2002; Povlsen, Olsen, & Ladelund, 2005).

Leininger (1991, 1995, 1998) refers to nursing as a transcultural phenomenon. She further submits that preparation in transcultural nursing is a prerequisite to working with diverse populations. Her Sunrise Model, discussed earlier in the chapter, enables the nurse to perform a cultural assessment or inquiry using the following concepts:

- *Worldview*—The client's perspective of his or her world and experiences
- *Ethnohistory*—Questions concerning place of origin and cultural legacy
- *Kinship and social factors*—Social and personal relationships, quality of support
- *Cultural values, beliefs*—Questions about values, beliefs, preferences, and traditions necessary to ensure holistic health care
- *Religion and spirituality*—Data regarding healing and comforting practices used during illness or losses
- *Technology*—Issues concerning the usefulness or hindrance of technologies
- *Politics and legal factors*—Legal issues that impact well-being
- *Education*—Data concerning educational level, and its importance in health care
- *Language and communication*—Involves language, linguistic competence, and language of choice
- *Professional and generic beliefs/practices*—Traditional Western medicine, folk medicine, or alternative or complementary health practices
- *General and specific nursing care*—Identify the meaning of quality nursing care within a sociocultural context (Leininger, 1991, 1995, 1998)

This cultural assessment model offers a comprehensive data gathering process through which the nurse garners a greater understanding of the client's needs and wishes. Questions posed during this process also convey concern and caring about the distinctiveness each client brings to the nurse–client encounter. As client advocates, nurses must communicate this information to the treatment planning team to ensure individualized diagnosis and interventions, and to advance positive clinical outcomes. Quality client advocacy and helping the client navigate complex health care systems also requires cultural competence.

Students, novices, and experienced nurses must develop knowledge that enables them to provide holistic health care across the life span. Paasche-Orlow (2004) asserts that integrating cultural competence into the medical curricula allows for an evaluation of the relationship between Western ethics and the ethics of cultural competence. Culturally competent nurses and other clinicians promote the following principles of cultural competence:

- Accept and appreciate the importance of culture in people's daily lives.
- Value cultural differences.
- Minimize cultural differences between the clinician and client.
- Embrace pluralism.
- Learn about the culture.
- Proactively accommodate differences.

To improve the quality of health care and clinical outcomes, the nurse must be able to communicate and understand fundamental differences among individuals from varied cultures, ethnicities, places of origin, and family backgrounds. These differences influence customs, wishes, preferences, and health care practices. Cultural competence advances autonomy, equitable health care, and collaborative nurse–client interactions while fostering trust and positive clinical outcomes. Although cultural competence is not a panacea, it fosters nurse–client relationships that convey empathy and a genuine responsiveness to client needs, wishes, preferences, and health care practices. True culturally sensitive or client-centered care involves performing an objective assessment, active shared decision making involving the client and family, and focusing on the client's physical, emotional, mental, and spiritual and religious needs (Leighton, 2005).

As already mentioned in this chapter, a lack of cultural competence or sensitivity undermines the provision of holistic health care, increases misdiagnoses, and results in inappropriate interventions and poor clinical outcomes. Approaching each client as an individual is essential to avoid missteps, embarrassment, and disrespect. Each person, regardless of ethnicity, culture, gender, or age, must be respected as an individual with his or her own attributes and needs. Nurses must assess and understand how beliefs, culture, gender, socialization, and values embody the client's experiences and perception of illness and health. Quality nurse–client interactions evolve through active listening, empathy, emotional support, and communication skills that enable the nurse to assess environments and communities in which the client lives as well as rituals, customs, and health practices unique to the client and family. Obtaining cultural competency is a lifelong process that evolves over a continuum (Cross et al., 1989) and is guided by the nurse's understanding of his or her own personal culture, values, and beliefs that vary from the client's. How the nurse adapts to these differences depends on the degree of self-awareness of biases and stereotyping, and his or her capacity and willingness to understand different cultures and integrate them into health care.

Disparities in health care have been extensively researched with primary foci on racial, ethnic, and socioeconomic inequities. Gender and generational or age-related disparities, particularly those affecting women and older adults, have been studied less. Results of disparities among women and older adults (Gurwitz et al., 2002; Jerant et al., 2004; Majeed & Cook, 1996; Ory, Kinney-Hoffman, Hawkins, Sanner, & Mockenhaupt, 2003) include hindering access to care, employing poor provider–client communication, deferring of specific diagnostic tests, and failing to implement evidence-based health care. Age-related and gender disparities, poor communication, ageism, and disrespect may contribute to poor clinical outcomes (American Cancer Society, 2002). Communication skills that ensure holistic, high-quality care of all clients, including individuals from diverse cultural and ethnic backgrounds, may improve health care (Lazare, Putnam, & Lipkin, 1995) across the life span.

Self-Awareness

A lengthy discussion of self-awareness is included in Chapters 1 and 2. Because self-awareness is a core component in all nurse–client interactions, a brief discussion is relevant at this time. Nurses can understand clients only as much as they understand themselves. The nurse's culture shapes personal values, beliefs, mores, customs, self-esteem, and self-worth and guides health practices and decision making. Everyone has "blind spots" or subjective lenses that compromise impartiality and hinder healthy nurse–client interactions.

Self-awareness is critical to cultural competence and requires acknowledging personal differences and their potential impact on nurse–client relationships. For instance, while working with a client from a different culture you notice he has a thick accent and you are unable to discern what he is saying. Rather than listening attentively and attempting to understand, you speak loudly and remark "I can't understand what you are saying." This response conveys a lack of empathy, disrespect, insensitivity, and an unwillingness to take the time to understand the client. What effect do you think this action has on the nurse–client relationship? Another example of a cultural difference is the client who does not make eye contact, which you interpret as negative or as low self-esteem. Is this really the basis of the poor eye contact? Or is a lack of or limited eye contact a common characteristic of the client's culture or ethnicity? Frequently, the nurse is unaware that her or his behaviors and communication methods, both verbal and nonnonverbal may convey the "wrong" or "inappropriate" message. Self-awareness also includes awareness of verbal and nonverbal means of communication, such as voice intonation, accent, gestures and facial expressions, touch, space, eye contact, and dress.

Assessing the individuality of every client's culture helps the nurse gain a clearer and more accurate understanding of his or her own culture, values, beliefs, mores, and customs. A willingness and ability to embrace the client's culture and ethnicity show respect toward the client and his or her family. According to researchers (Giger & Davidhizar, 2004; Leininger, 1995; Purnell & Paulanka, 2003), nurses must assess clients according to several cultural phenomena to ensure cultural competence:

- Communication styles
- Time
- Space
- Social organization

Communication Style

Communication is essential for survival. It is the means of understanding self and others and forming interpersonal relationships and seeking help. Verbal and nonverbal communication varies among individuals, cultures, families, and communities. Encounters with diverse groups require the nurse to understand communication patterns, both verbal and nonverbal; language; and the social context of values, beliefs, and health practices. When assessing the meaning of verbal and nonverbal communication it is imperative to understand that communication is a complex process that involves active listening and interpreting an array of behaviors simultaneously. People communicate through facial gestures, voice intonation, dress, grooming and hygiene, and posture. Several questions may be helpful in evaluating verbal and nonverbal communication:

- What is socially and culturally acceptable to the client, family, and community?
- What behaviors are offensive or convey insincerity?
- How do I appear to others?
- Does the client understand what I am trying to communicate?

- Are my verbal cues congruent with nonverbal cues?
- Am I using words or communication the client clearly understands?
- When should I consider using an interpreter?

It behooves the nurse to understand communication patterns, both verbal and nonverbal, that are distinct to each client. Equally important is self-awareness of our own cultural communication patterns and how they may conflict with the client's. If eye contact is an important or "normal" feature of the nurse's communication pattern and the client maintains little or avoids eye contact, it is imperative for the nurse to recognize this may be "normal" rather than "abnormal" to ensure the client's needs are met. Words or symbols are also important communication tools. A client's physical markings, such as facial scars or tattoos, may conflict with the nurse's beliefs, but must be understood as part of a cultural ritual or tribal marking. What do these markings represent? Facial markings may communicate the client's tribal affiliation or ethnicity. This is an important feature and communication pattern of countries with numerous ethnic groups. Knowledge of rituals, physical markings, and customs permits the nurse to approach each encounter objectively and provide culturally sensitive care. The more knowledge the nurse possesses concerning diverse cultures, ethnicities, and the meaning of rituals, the greater chance he or she has of establishing rapport and trust—necessary features of quality and effective nurse–client relationships.

Physical grooming and hygiene must also be assessed within a social context to determine if poor hygiene represents poor functional status or customs and rituals unique to diverse groups. Although a lack of physical grooming and poor hygiene, or certain mouth and body odors, such as garlic, curry, or tobacco, may be offensive to the nurse, it is imperative to employ a culturally sensitive approach before ascribing the behavior as pathological or abnormal. In the event this behavior is not part of the client's culture, the nurse must further assess for a serious physical or mental health problem.

Establishing rapport using open communication and a nonjudgmental approach is pivotal in creating helping relationships. Knowledge of how diverse client populations communicate is also important. The client may perceive the nurse who is talkative, uses medical jargon, and is detailed oriented as offensive or disrespectful. For instance, the Native American client may prefer less talk and be comfortable with silence. In this situation the nurse needs to speak less, listen more, and respect silence. In addition, using humor or assuming that certain types of body language, such as eye contact, are common across cultures may be detrimental to helping relationships.

Humor may be perceived as ridiculing, demeaning, or wearing a mask unless trust and a helping relationship have been established (Maples et al., 2001). However, in situations where trust and helping relationships have been established, researchers submit that humor and laughter are an important communication tool in many cultures, including the Native American culture. Knowledge of humor and its impact on helping relationships, particularly within the Native American culture, fosters a greater understanding of the example client's experiences. It can be used to reduce stress and tension and strengthen the client's spiritual and religious experience (Dean, 2003; Lincoln, 1993). Wittiness may also be a way to convey a serious message within a humorous context. Knowledge of humor within the Native American culture enables the nurse to use humor appropriately within the social context of nurse–client relationships (Dean; Lincoln; Nilsen & Nilsen, 2000).

Improving quality of care across the life span requires client empowerment. Health education is an integral part of that empowerment. Health education and information about drug trials and evidence-based treatment must be disseminated through various means including non-English-speaking media, culturally based media, the Internet, and religious and community organizations to help diverse groups access health care and dialogue more proficiently with the nurse and other clinicians.

As nurses interact with individuals from diverse cultures, it is imperative to focus on the individual's needs and accept variations, such as gender, age, socioeconomic and education levels, value preferences, sexual orientation, health practices, and perceptions of health and illness. This approach ensures holistic and individualized care and facilitates positive clinical outcomes. Patience, respect for differences, dignity, and positive regard for the client's uniqueness must always be the focus of nurse–client encounters.

Time

Time is one of the most important aspects of communication. Its meaning varies among cultures and frequently conflicts with the nurse's view of time. For example, some cultures view time within a present and future orientation, whereas others focus solely on present time. Expectations about punctuality are also linked to time references; one client may be 30 minutes late for an appointment and another may be early or on time. Assessing the meaning of time helps the nurse determine the significance of lateness, which may differ among the clients. Lateness may not indicate a lack of motivation or unwillingness to participate in treatment; it may reflect the client's normal daily patterns, in which timeliness may be less significant.

Concerns about lateness must be communicated effectively to reduce misunderstanding and conflicts and ensure quality nurse–client interactions. The following scenario demonstrates how the nurse can address this issue:

Mary is a 34-year-old client who consistently comes late to her diabetic education class. Each time she arrives late, other group members express concerns about the disruption. Despite efforts to address this issue in the diabetic education class, the nurse has been unsuccessful in having Mary appear on time. At today's meeting she asks Mary to meet her after class.

Nurse: Mary, as you know, I wanted to meet with you about your lateness and its impact on other group members.

Mary: I don't understand why everyone is so upset. I've only been 10 minutes late each time.

Nurse: I understand that 10 minutes may be insignificant to you, but it is important me and the other group members. You are an important member of the class and when you come in late, it disrupts the meeting.

Mary: I didn't know I was that important that others noticed me coming in late.

Nurse: Everyone is important, including you. When you come in late members may perceive it as disrespectful or that you don't care about them or the class.

Mary: I do care. I didn't realize coming in late was such a big deal. It's nice that others value me so much. I will come to the meeting on time next week. Thanks.

Although the nurse did not focus on cultural issues involving time, the client's perception of time differed from the nurse's and group members'. Left unresolved, this issue may have had a negative impact on member relationships and the quality of the class. Clearly, the client needs to participate in the diabetic education class, but her lateness had to be addressed in a timely manner to ensure access to quality health care and positive clinical outcomes for all group members. Addressing time and other culturally related health matters requires assertive communication skills to convey empathy and understanding, but firm limit setting ensures the rights of all clients to access health education and clinical care. Apart from imparting information, the nurse also displayed respect and understanding, and described timeliness as an expectation of all members.

Purnell and Paulanka (2003) suggest the following questions to assess time or temporal relationships:

- Is the client primarily past-, present-, or future-oriented?
- How does the client perceive the past, present, or future?
- How does the client define time frames? Is the individual expected to be on time or punctual for his or her job or appointments?

Answers to these questions help the nurse understand the meaning of time for the client and family. The nurse needs to specify the importance of being on time for appointments to reduce misunderstandings between the client and nurse (Purnell & Paulanka, 2003).

Space

Anthropologist Edward T. Hall in his seminal publication, *The Hidden Dimension* (1966), explicated distinct difference perception among various cultures. In this classic book he described four distinct distance zones maintained by healthy, middle-class Americans. Hall recognized that perceptions of distance zones vary among cultures. The aim of delineating these four distance zones was to increase the understanding of how they differ among various cultural and socioeconomic groups. Based on his explanation, he asserted that one's comfort zones are contingent on how one feels about the person they are interacting with at the time of the encounter. As more and more nurses interact with each other and various cultures it is helpful to understand the impact of one's own culture on how comfortable one feels with others at any given encounter. Awareness of the client's need to maintain an acceptable distance facilitates a sense of security and acceptance. (See a comprehensive discussion of space in Chapter 1.)

The four distance zones are:

1. *Intimate distance/close range*—The presence of another person is obvious during intimate encounters. This is demonstrated in love-making, hugging, contact sports, or kissing a loved one or friend. It also occurs when the nurse performs activities of daily living, checks vital signs, or assists the client with meals.
2. *Personal distance*—Enables the nurse to discuss personal interests at arm's length distance. This ranges from 1½ to 4 feet. A handshake is an example of something taking place in personal space. This is also demon-

strated when the nurse does health education groups with clients and families.

3. *Social distance*—often referred to as close distance. This ranges from 4 to 12 feet. This distance involves minimum physical contact and occurs during a staff meeting or teleconference, interactions with a bank teller, or in a waiting room.

4. *Public distance*—This ranges from 12 to 25 feet or more and there is minimal eye contact. This takes place when walking through an airport or passing someone on the road or public speaking events. It allows for easy escape or defensive action. There is mutual respect to maintain distance and remain strangers. (Hall 1966, 1989)

Appreciation of **cultural space** is critical to establishing effective nurse–client communication and individualized care. Leininger (1995) defines cultural space as "variation of cultures in the use of body, visual, territorial, and interpersonal distance to others" (p. 77). Self-awareness concerning space and understanding its potential impact on interactions with diverse populations are critical. This extends beyond nurse–client relationships to include interactions with colleagues, families, and communities. Knowledge of cultural space helps the nurse create a comfortable distance that allays anxiety, facilitates helping interactions and appropriate responses based on space distinction. When physical and emotional closeness are not endorsed or practiced by a culture, family, or community, moving close to someone engenders distress, anxiety, and distrust, which are major barriers to effective communication.

Failure to assess and respect space differences or "comfort zones" can have a detrimental effect on interpersonal relationships. For instance, the nurse who is "touchy feely" or likes to hug and touch may be perceived as intrusive and "attacking" to some individuals. In some cases when touching is necessary, such as performing vital signs and bathing, the nurse should ask permission, provide an explanation for the touching, and maintain a professional demeanor during the encounter. Violation of the client's space can also increase nonadherence to treatment and result in poor clinical outcomes. Disrespecting the client's need for distance increases anxiety and distress, which may result in violence or aggression to "protect self." These reactions are more likely to occur in situations in which the client has a history of trauma or is distrustful due to disorganized thought processes, altered sensory perceptions, and developmental or gender factors. In comparison, others may value physical closeness and feel very comfortable with the nurse being in their personal space. Despite the client's comfort with physical closeness, the nurse must maintain an appropriate distance to ensure personal safety, establish clear boundaries, and reduce miscommunication of nonverbal cues. Insight into cultural space is pivotal during interactions with clients, families, and colleagues to ensure clear and safe boundaries beneficial to healing interpersonal relationships.

Social Organization

Giger and Davidhizar (2004) describe social organizations as processes in which the family functions. This concept is similar to other family therapy theories, which define family systems as social institutions with mutually sustaining qualities (Boyd-Franklin, 1989; Satir, 1967). Families transmit culture, values, norms, traditions, communication patterns, language, and religious and spiritual beliefs and establish boundaries between subsystems. They also define the roles and functions of family membership, boundaries between generations, and expression of emotions, health practices, and health-seeking behaviors. Working with clients and their families requires a basic understanding of how the family functions within the social context of culture.

Communication patterns, time, space, and social organization have different meanings in various cultures. Nurses must assess their meaning and impact on nurse–client interactions. The complexity of communication across cultures emphasizes the importance of cultural competence and a willingness to understand the individuality each client brings to the nurse–client encounter.

CULTURE AND COMMUNICATION ACROSS THE LIFE SPAN

A plethora of evidence indicates that racial and ethnic inequities in health care that are related to the quality of the clinician–client relationship contribute to health disparities, reduce access to care, breech continuity of care, reduce client satisfaction, and produce poor clinical outcomes (IOM, 2003; Stewart, 1995). It also shows the importance of cultural competence and a lifelong willingness to value and appreciate diversity and devise interventions that ensure holistic care. Regardless of developmental stage, individualized and holistic principles must guide the nurse in seeking to understand and communicate with diverse populations whose beliefs, values, wishes, and health care practices differ from mainstream Western society. This approach must be used in all client interactions because everyone has a culture and is part of several subcultures, such as age or generation, gender, socioeconomic status, geographic location, religion, physical disability, education level, and sexual orientation. Culturally sensitive and individualized nursing care requires a communication process that integrates these variables across the health care continuum, beginning with the assessment process.

Assessment Process

Leininger's Sunrise Model (1991) provides guidance in performing a client-centered and holistic assessment of clients, families, and communities. These principles are designed to respect the uniqueness each client brings to the nurse–client relationship. Salient points from her theory include:

- Use active listening skills to understand the client's perspective, sociocultural factors, linguistics, and social and environmental context.
- Employ communication free of jargon, but unique to the client and family's needs.
- Focus on the client's experience, health practices, wishes, beliefs, and preferences.
- Avoid use of personal beliefs, values, and preferences, especially if they differ from the client's.
- Encourage the client to discuss his or her life experiences, expectations, and needs through various means including storytelling and cultural icons, poems, photographs, songs, rituals, and dress.
- Utilize open-ended questions to understand the unique richness each client brings to the nurse–client relationship.
- Maintain confidentiality.

Leininger (1995) describes the assessment process as a dynamic creative journey and meaningful discovery process that enables the nurse to collaborate with the client and family and expand his or her insight into the client's experiences. During illness, some clients become more isolated and passive; others may become more demanding and have difficulty coping with health-related concerns. Understanding culture and its potential role in the client's experiences can be accomplished when the nurse:

- Assesses and provides staff education concerning health beliefs, values, norms, traditions, and the meaning of health and illness within a given culture
- Learns as much as possible to grasp the meaning of how the client understands, communicates, and responds to stress and illness

- Assesses the impact of the client's illness on functional status and emotional and physical status
- Integrates the client's cultural needs into a comprehensive and holistic plan of care
- Formulates assessment approaches that elicit client perceptions about their illness, health practices, and expectations of treatment
- Uses culturally sensitive communication to establish nurse–client healing relationships
- Engages the client in active participation in shared decision making

A leading challenge of today's nurse is distinguishing behavioral responses and communication patterns unique to diverse groups from abnormal behavior. Overall, the assessment process affords the nurse opportunities to understand the client within a social dimension impacted by culture, values, beliefs, traditions, and norms. Collectively, this approach ensures individualized and holistic health care and facilitates quality outcomes across the life span. As a mediator of health care, the nurse is also responsible for communicating assessment data to the interdisciplinary team to ensure data gathered during the assessment process is transmitted accurately to ensure a factual diagnosis, appropriate treatment planning, and positive clinical outcomes. Equally important is evaluation of the health care system and its attitude towards diversity and shared decision making.

Children and Adolescents

Never before has there been a greater need to assess and value culture across the life span and its potential impact on the care of children and their families. Caring for the ill child is a family affair that involves parents and other family members including grandparents and siblings. Seriously or critically ill children of all cultures place a tremendous emotional and physical burden on the child and family. Coping with this situation is often overtaxing to the family and generates strong emotional reactions, such as anger, sadness, depression, agitation, and helplessness. Efforts to assess their needs, mitigate frustration, and understand health-related behaviors are imperative. Questions to ask the family include:

- What is the primary language spoken by adults in the home?
- How big (extended) is the family?
- What type of residence does the family live in?

- Are there any smokers living at home?
- What educational level have the parents completed?
- What are your current support systems and financial resources?

Answers to these questions can be used to guide the nurse in the assessment and treatment planning process. Open communication with the child and family about basic and complex health care needs imparts knowledge and conveys respect and dignity. The more the nurse understands and appreciates the sociocultural factors and unique qualities of the child, family, and community, the more likely she or he can help the client navigate the health care system and ensure individualized health care.

Every culture practices customs and traditions and values its children within a social context that provides for their basic needs, safety, and emotional and physical support to ensure self-preservation for future generations (Cross et al., 1989). Virginia Satir (1967), a renowned family therapist, described a family as a social institution bonded by mutual interests, beliefs, and values. Within this social context, traditions, beliefs, communication patterns, and norms are molded, nurtured, developed, and transmitted to children and perpetuated across generations through parental styles, communication patterns and language, and expression and value of emotions, with the ultimate goal of the child becoming a healthy adult.

Communication and language are an integral part of culture. Through verbal and nonverbal gestures, such as frowning, smiling, grimacing, or glaring, the child learns to communicate feelings, thoughts, emotions, and behaviors. Parental modeling provides the structure; parent–child interactions instill language and validate the meaning and appropriateness of gestures and verbal communication.

Working with infants and children requires an understanding of the family's communication patterns, language, socialization, eating patterns, dress, and means of conveying emotions, feelings, and behaviors. The nurse must respect and build upon the child, family, and community culture and their strengths. Assessing family strengths enables the nurse to use them as the basis of the assessment process to diagnose, shore up their confidence and competence for active participation in shared decision making, and establish optimal clinical outcomes. Active nurse–client dialogue in the shared decision-making process is crucial. It increases family involvement through open communication, health education, and treatment planning. Higher client satisfaction and positive clinical outcomes have been associated with communicating prognostic information to families of critically ill clients (LeClaire, Oakes, & Weinert, 2005).

Cultural competence also requires sensitivity to the uniqueness of the parent–child interactions, customs, rituals, religious and spiritual needs, preferences, and developmental needs and wishes. Learning as much as possible about the youth and family's culture is important to be able to appraise their experiences. Equally significant is a thorough assessment of family roles and relationships, including siblings, grandparents, aunts, uncles, and other relatives. Strengthening the nurse–client relationship with both the child and family promotes cultural competence as well as identification and implementation of holistic care. Through cultural competence the nurse can focus on family strengths and positive characteristics, and rid him- or herself of biases and stereotypes. Ultimately, cultural competence enables the nurse to elicit distinct information unique to the client to make accurate diagnoses, negotiate acceptable treatment goals, and develop and implement client-centered interventions. As a result, cultural competence increases client and family satisfaction, expands client involvement, and facilitates positive clinical outcomes.

CRITICAL THINKING QUESTION

You are caring for a young Hispanic child who has recently been hospitalized for an acute asthma attack. During your initial encounter with the child, you notice his mother has limited English proficiency. Knowing the importance of working with parents caring for sick children, what is the most correct approach to this situation?

a. Ask one of the Cuban nurses to interpret or work with the mother.

b. Assess her language proficiency or preferred language through an interpreter.

c. Wait until one of the child's English-speaking relatives visits.

d. Find Spanish literature to facilitate communication.

It is imperative to assess and evaluate the family's language proficiency rather than assuming that all Hispanic cultures speak the same language (as in choice a). Asking a Cuban nurse to interpret the client's needs suggests that all Spanish-speaking individuals share the same cultural values, beliefs, and background. This assumption may be disrespectful to the child, family, and nurse. Involving an interpreter (choice b) is very helpful not only to evaluate language and facilitate client-centered nursing care, but also to ensure confidentiality and to gather an accurate account of the child or family's experience, which is sometimes not afforded by family interpreters (choice c). Waiting until an English-speaking relative visits the child also displays a lack of cultural sensitivity, particularly if the nurse is unaware of when this might occur. Also, families frequently prefer non-family members as interpreters, especially for personal matters they do not want shared with the family. Finding Spanish literature to facilitate communication (as in choice d) indicates a lack of understanding about language and communication within a defined culture. First of all, what type of literature are you referring to and how will it help you establish a relationship with the client's mother with limited English proficiency? Each family member must be treated as an individual. Spanish literature infers literature is appropriate for all Spanish-speaking and English-limited individuals.

Gender Sensitivity Considerations (Women)

Women's satisfaction with clinicians is more likely to be tied to continuity of care and quality of health education than is men's satisfaction (Weisman et al., 2000). Research shows that women are more likely to receive more information, ask questions, and experience more shared decision making than men (Kaplan, Gandek, Greenfield, Rogers, & Ware, 1995; Street, Gordon, Ward, Krupat, & Kravitz, 2005). Likewise, several studies indicate female physicians are more likely to convey empathy, make inquiries, and participate in shared decision making than male physicians (Roter, Hall, & Aoki, 2002; Street et al., 2005; van den Brink-Muinen, Bensing, & Kerssens, 1998). Regardless of gender, quality nurse–client interactions that foster shared decision making are an integral component of health care across the life span.

Women's health care issues encompass a broad range of health-related concerns, including communication difficulties with clinicians. Reproductive health, heart disease, diabetes, obesity, lung cancer, and HIV and AIDS are a few issues confronting women across the life span. Empowering women to make informed, confident, and competent shared decision making is key to identifying gender-related health issues and implementing interventions that ensure holistic health care. Similar to all clients, culture, socioeconomic status, age, education level, and linguistics play a key role in framing health care issues and nurse–client relationships. Cain (2001) notes two assumptions about women:

- Women want access to quality health care and the best care possible.
- Women will filter health practices and health education through cultural and emotional filters.

She further expressed concerns about the plight of rural women of all ages, shaped by geographic isolation, socioeconomic status, language, educational and cultural barriers, a higher incidence of domestic violence, greater distance from health care providers, and closed societies in which health ideas are slow to disseminate. Consequently, mistrust of health care providers challenges the nurse to establish trust, assess the meaning of health and illness, and use active listening skills to discern what the client believes are the essentials of good health care and acceptable clinical outcomes. Communication with women from rural areas must be deliberate and methodical while integrating their preferences, needs, customs, and health practices. Involving women in health care decisions, valuing cultural and gender preferences, and providing health education are essential elements of quality care. Collectively, shared decision making and gender-focused health care increase client satisfaction, confidence and competence and promote adherence to treatment, and contribute to positive clinical outcomes.

Researchers contend that a widening quality gap exists between women's wishes and values and their primary health care, particularly among women of lower socioeconomic status and urban groups (O'Malley & Forrest, 2002). A growing awareness of health care disparities for women makes it clear that nurses must seek opportunities to form quality interactions and address issues unique to women across the life span. Older persons, especially older women, often believe their health care needs are inadequately assessed during encounters with health care providers. Generational and socialization issues play key roles in older women asserting themselves and actively engaging themselves in shared decision making. Educating and empowering older women to understand their right to participate in treatment is crucial to advancing their needs, values, and choices (Roberts, 2004).

The following scenario demonstrates a nurse–client situation involving health education and assertive communication:

Mrs. Ellis, a 78-year-old client, is seen in ambulatory care after a left hip replacement. She expresses concern that her pain medication is not working as well as it did shortly after surgery. She also reports concern about discussing this with her physician for fear he will think she is addicted to pain medication.

Nurse: Good morning, Mrs. Ellis. I see this is your first visit since your surgery. How are you doing?

Client: Well, I am still having difficulty sleeping due to pain in my left hip.

Nurse: Is your pain limited to bedtime?

Client: Yes, that's when I notice it the most.

Nurse: What makes it worse at nighttime?

Client: I guess because I take my medication in the morning and stay busy. But my husband tells me I toss and turn a lot at night.

Nurse: On a scale of 1 to 10 (1 = minimal pain and 10 = severe pain), how much pain do you have at night?

Client: About 8.

Nurse: What stops you from taking pain medication before you go to bed?

Client: I don't want to get hooked on drugs.

Nurse: As your doctor explained before surgery, pain medication is necessary to help you heal and promote rest. Obviously, taking one pain pill per day is not enough. Let's talk to your physician and discuss ways to manage your pain more effectively.

Client: He might get mad at me, and I don't want to bother him with minor things.

Nurse: Pain control is a serious matter, and you have a right to control your pain. If you take the medication as ordered the chances of becoming addicted to it are minimal.

Client: You mean Dr. Okon won't get upset if I bring this up today?

Nurse: No—in fact he expects you to report these things so he can better manage your pain. Unless you discuss it with him, how can he help?

Client: I don't want to be a burden or complain too much.

Nurse: Dr. Okon wants to hear your concerns and you are not a burden. Let's see him now.

This scenario demonstrates how to empower an older female client who minimizes her pain and puts concerns of what the physician will say or do over her personal well-being, comfort, and health. Through patience, respect, empathy, and trust the nurse provides health education about pain management and the importance of discussing it with her physician. The process depicted in the dialogue would be strengthened by timely and adequate documentation of the nurse's conversation with the client and verbally communicating their conversation to the client's physician, to ensure her concerns are clearly understood.

Families

Working with families requires strong communication skills and an astute understanding of communication patterns, problem-solving processes, coping styles, strengths, and relevant norms, rules, traditions, roles, and structure. Learning about families requires patience and trusting relationships that encourage members to discuss how tasks and roles are determined. Whether family rules are guided by generational traditions or contemporary influences, the roles of men and women vary among cultures and ethnic groups. Despite the changing roles of men and women in Western societies, many cultural expectations are tied to traditions and passed from generation to generation. In many cultures men are expected to be in control, whereas women are expected to be compliant and acquiescent (Zielke-Nadkarni, 2003). Regardless, nurses must understand and respect family structure, assess communication patterns and interactions, determine the quality of member support, and recognize the influence of their own culture and perception of family on the client's. Families often play key roles as caregivers of the very young and very old. Enlisting them in the client's care is often crucial to how the client manages illness and health within the health care system and community.

Equally important is gathering data about religious or spiritual practices, family solidarity in the community, value conflict (which emerges when one's personal religious or spiritual beliefs differ from one's family of origin), socioeconomic status, and education level. The client's basic beliefs about reality and truth or worldview are associated with his or her cultural, religious, and spiritual perspectives and have enormous implications for clinical outcomes (Warren, 2003). For instance, if a person with a serious or chronic disease believes in fatalism or his or her worldview is that his or her fate is predetermined and there is little motivation to adhere to treatment. Questions about perceptions of causation of disease or illness and health practices, which often include folklore medicine (e.g., *curanderos*); alternative or complementary therapies, such as herbal remedies; and the client and family's understanding of treatment options must be an integral part of the nursing process (Fernandez et al., 2004; Padilla et al., 2001). Exploring the role of secrecy, particularly when the client is terminally ill and the family does not want him or her to know, and its meaning must be addressed to ensure the client's rights are not violated. Failure to identify and address these issues contributes to health disparities and poor clinical outcomes. Students, novices, and experienced nurses must be able to join the family and establish working relationships to assess the needs of the client, family, and community. Relationships with the family are critical to shared decision making, building confidence, treatment planning, and the implementation of holistic health care.

Discerning the client's role and functions within the family is also important. Some families encourage individuality, whereas others are reluctant to encourage it. In the latter case, problem solving is more likely to occur within the nuclear and extended family. Recognizing the impact of these dynamics on the nurse–client relationship and incorporating their wishes into care planning is paramount. Traditionally, when working with clients, the spouse or other members of the nuclear family assist in decision making and actively participate in health care. In families where problem solving occurs between the nuclear and extended families the situation may vary and be difficult to assess. Nurses must refrain from assuming the former family dynamics or interactions occur in all families. Regardless, determining the client's wishes, preferences, and needs must guide the nurse in determining the role of the family and community in addressing health care problems. Nurses must adhere to federal guidelines, regulations, and ethical principles when dealing with privacy issues and discussing the client's problems with the family.

The following nurse–client encounter demonstrates the potential impact of culture on interactions with families:

Mrs. Bartinelli, an 80-year-old woman, recently was diagnosed with colon cancer and the family has been informed of the prognosis. During morning rounds, her oldest son asks the nurse not to share the prognosis with the client because it would be harmful to her.

Mr. Bartinelli: Are you my mother's nurse today?

Nurse: Yes.

Mr. Bartinelli: Please don't tell my mother about her condition.

Nurse: What do you mean?

Mr. Bartinelli: I don't believe she can cope with such bad news.

Nurse: Mr. Bartinelli, I respect your concerns, but the decision to discuss your mother's prognosis has to be a team decision. Have you discussed your concerns with her physician?

Mr. Bartinelli: No, but I plan to discuss it with her.

Nurse: I know how difficult this is for you and your family. I will call your mother's doctor and inform her of the family's concerns to determine the best approach to this situation.

Mr. Bartinelli: I am very worried, but I trust her doctor will make the best decision for my mother and the family.

This scenario demonstrates the importance of active listening skills and effective communication to assess the needs of the client's son. It also demonstrates the cultural sensitivity since some families protect loved ones from "bad" news because they often fear that if they tell the client he or she will become hopeless and give up. Equally important is addressing the client's right to information concerning her prognosis and treatment considerations. The nurse was willing to hear and understand the son's concerns, and her willingness to follow up with the client's physician and interdisciplinary team displayed cultural sensitivity. Ethical dilemmas often occur when the family's needs supersede the client's.

Older Adulthood

Working with older adults requires sensitivity to an array of factors unique to this age group. Cultural, socioeconomic, and generational issues; health-related problems; and literacy impact how nurses communicate with older adults. Nursing strategies must center on respect, dignity, and appreciation of the wisdom that comes with longevity as well as an understanding of client values, sociocultural needs, wishes, preferences, and health practices. This is particularly significant when the client's cultural background and generational issues differ from the nurse's. Similar to other age groups, trust and helping relationships evolve from effective communication skills that convey respect, patience, acceptance, understanding, and support. A failure to integrate these factors into nurse–client relationships can have detrimental effects, such as mistrust, alienation from the nurse and health care, and further health care disparities. As society ages and nurses interact more often with older clients, it is imperative to link culture, ethnicity, gender, language, communication patterns, education level, socioeconomic status, and age-related factors into the nursing process to ensure equitable and quality health care for this population.

As previously discussed, health disparities among culturally diverse groups also occur for older adults, particularly in situations involving diagnostic studies, procedures, and appropriate treatment (Cooper-Patrick et al., 1999; IOM, 2001; Welch, Teno, & Mor, 2005). Health disparities also are linked to communication or linguistic differences, which may prevent the nurse from understanding the client's needs, wishes, and preferences; imparting health education; and providing emotional support. A cross-sectional, retrospective national survey that compared the end-of-life medical care experienced by African American and white patients and their families (surrogate, $n = 1,447$) demonstrated persistent health care disparities (Welch et al., 2005). Symptom management, informed decision making, individual and family support, coordination of services, and financial impact were addressed in the survey. Findings from the study indicated family members of African Americans were less apt than those of whites to communicate that their loved ones' needs were met. Researchers also submit that health care continues into end-of-life issues, particularly concerning communication and addressing family needs, such as home care patterns and financial support (Welch et al.). Implications for nursing practice from these data and other studies include the necessity to assess the unique needs of the older adult and family members to ensure holistic needs are addressed during end-of-life and other health-related situations. Communication about procedures, informed consent, advance directives, and health education are critical components of transcultural care (Foy, Penninx, Shumaker, Messier, & Pahor, 2005).

An aging society and changing demographics require nursing competence that employs holistic strategies. Individualized nursing care requires open communication that integrates the individuality of each client and includes preferences, wishes, traditions, perceptions of illness and health, language, and health practice. Involving the client and family in decision making and providing individualized health education affords holistic health care and improves clinical outcomes.

SUMMARY

Transcultural nursing care must transcend cultural barriers while ensuring respect and valuing the differences of each client. Current health disparities challenge nurses to provide individualized care within a pluralistic society that focuses primarily on biomedicine. Addressing the health care needs of diverse cultural groups requires looking beyond Western medicine and incorporating health practices based on the client's preferences, wishes, and customs. Equally important is developing quality nurse–client relationships and communication skills that convey empathy and respect, ensure dignity, and open communication channels to assess and understand the meaning of client experiences and responses to illness. Helping and collaborative relationships advance client needs through complex health care systems, and increase client satisfaction and positive clinical care. Cultural competence is the venue in which these actions occur.

Cultural competence evolves through nurse–client relationships and is a conduit that allows the nurse to use each encounter with the client, family, and community to grasp the meaning of the values, beliefs, preferences, traditions, and mores that guide communication patterns, coping styles, and perceptions of health and illness. Nursing competence transcends cultural competence because each client must be addressed as an individual with unique qualities, responses, abilities, and strengths. Nursing competence also means avoiding stereotyping or assuming certain behaviors based on gender, race, culture, ethnicity, or age. A willingness and capacity to learn about individuals regardless of social or cultural context is the core of cultural competence. This process is governed by the ability to recognize how cultural competence shapes opinions of others. Self-awareness is a guiding force of cultural competence. With maturity and experience, students, novices, and experienced nurses can become proficient in assessing the needs of all clients to ensure culturally sensitive health care across the life span.

SUGGESTIONS FOR CLINICAL AND EXPERIENTIAL ACTIVITIES

1. Go to the National Center for Cultural Competence Web site at http://gucchd.georgetown.edu/nccc/orgselfassess.html#benefits, and discuss your self-assessment findings in class, include the following.
   a. Assess the degree in which you effectively address the needs and preferences of culturally and linguistically diverse groups.
   b. Establish meaningful nurse–client and key community stakeholders relationships.
   c. Identify and promote personal growth that enhances your ability to deliver individualized and culturally sensitive competent health care.
   d. Provide a forum to give honest statements about your level of awareness, knowledge, and skills related to cultural and linguistic competence.

2. Develop a case study of a culture different from your own. Assess their traditions and rituals and their impact on illness and health, and present your findings to the class.

3. Seek out a shadowing experience with a bilingual or trilingual clinician to discuss important communication strategies, including using an interpreter, to establish a relationship and work with a client with limited English proficiency.

4. Seek clinical experiences that focus on generational or developmental factors associated with aging and older adults.

5. Volunteer at your local area Agency for Aging and meet with staff and residents to discuss community and social services available to older women of diverse cultural, racial, and ethnic backgrounds.

6. Participate in scenarios or role-playing to assess stereotyping and culturally insensitive communication and relationships.

END-OF-CHAPTER QUESTIONS

1. Mr. Hernandez, a 54-year-old client, is seen in the primary care clinic with a diagnosis of Type II diabetes. During the course of the visit he insists on seeing a male nurse because he needs to discuss a personal concern. What is the most appropriate response?
   a. May I ask why you want to see a male nurse?
   b. How can I help? I can help just as well as a male nurse.
   c. Just a minute, I will get a male nurse to assist you.
   d. We don't have any male nurses on duty today.

2. Ms. Marshall, a 40-year-old woman, inquires about her upcoming routine mammogram. Considering gender-related health care issues, which of the following might you expect from her?
   a. Tell me more about the examination, including risks.
   b. Do you have pamphlets that explain this procedure?
   c. Can you suggest any Internet sites that explain the procedure?
   d. All of the above.

3. Health education is an important nursing intervention. Mr. Jones and his wife are attending a health education class on "Managing Hypertension." Which question demonstrates transcultural nursing care?
   a. Do you like fried foods?
   b. Do you eat a lot of salt?
   c. What kind of over-the-counter medications do you take?
   d. All of the above.

4. Mr. Jessup is an 86-year-old veteran seeking follow-up treatment for coronary artery disease. As his nurse, which of the following depicts cultural competence?
   a. Mr. Jessup, I need to take your blood pressure; which arm do you prefer?
   b. Let me help you honey.
   c. Do you want me to read these instructions for you?
   d. How often does your family let your drive alone?

5. Jon, a 12-year-old boy who speaks fluent English, recently has been hospitalized for acute appendicitis. While checking his temperature you notice his mother offering him herbal tea. You question her about the drink and she gets upset. You also discover she speaks very little English. What is the most appropriate response?
   a. Use a nonthreatening and supportive approach.
   b. Ask the youth to communicate to his mother that he is not supposed to have fluids.
   c. Ask an interpreter to explain her son's situation and current treatment.
   d. All of the above.

6. Cultural competence is synonymous with nursing competence.
   a. True
   b. False

7. Which of the following questions represents Worldview in Leininger's Transcultural Sunrise Model?
   a. What do you call your illness?
   b. Tell me how your illness is impacting your life.
   c. What can I do to make your stay more comfortable?
   d. Explain health practices you use to manage stress.

Answers

7. a
6. True
5. d
4. a
3. c
2. d
1. c

Research Study 4–1

Title: Barriers Influencing the Success of Racial and Ethnic Minority Students in Nursing Programs. Gardner, J. (2005). *Journal of Transcultural Nursing, 16,* 155–162.

Purpose: The author sought to document the role of culture, social integration, and educator characteristics of minority student nurses' perspectives of their experiences in predominantly white nursing programs. The author sought to understand their perspectives as a venue to help nurse educators meet the students' educational needs and increase graduation among minority students.

Method: The author used a phenomenology approach to explore how human beings interpret an experience and transform the experience to awareness. This phenomenological qualitative study explored the experience of being a minority student in a predominantly white nursing program. **Design.** A quantitative study of 15 minority nursing students' experiences while enrolled in a predominantly white nursing program was conducted. Comprehensive interviews were conducted using a semistructured approach guided by open-ended and probing questions to elicit feelings and experiences. Participants ranged from 27 to 47 years of age; 13 were female and 2 were male. Specific student cultural backgrounds were 3 East Indian, 2 Hispanic, 2 Hmong (Laotian), 2 African American, 2 Nigerian, 1 Filipino, 1 Nepalese, 1 Chinese, and 1 Vietnamese.

Results/Findings: Eight themes emerged from the interviews, which were not unique to being a foreign- or American-born minority nursing student. Data analysis reflected participants' perceptions of the faculty, peers, and nursing school experience. The eight themes were loneliness and isolation, differences, absence of acknowledgment of individuality from teachers, peers' lack of understanding and knowledge about cultural differences, desiring support from teachers, coping with insensitivity and discrimination, determination to build a better future, and overcoming obstacles.

Implications for Nurses: As mentioned in this chapter, nurses are challenged to work with and provide health care to diverse cultures. Cultural competence or sensitivity extends beyond students or nurses to their clients and includes peers and colleagues. Self-awareness is crucial to understanding personal values, beliefs, and perceptions of self and others. The author stresses the importance of being empathetic and sensitive, and mentoring students from diverse cultural and ethnic backgrounds. Role modeling these behaviors provides a learning experience for all students and nurses.

REFERENCES

American Association of Colleges of Nursing. (2001). Issue bulletin: Effective strategies for increasing diversity in nursing programs. Retrieved September 17, 2005, from http://www.aacn.nche.edu/Publications/issues/dec01.htm

American Cancer Society. (2002). Breast cancer facts and figures: 2001–2002. Retrieved September 17, 2005, from http://www.cancer.org/docroot/STT/content/STT_1x_Breast_Cancer_Facts_and_Figures_2001–2002.asp

Boyd-Franklin, N. (1989). *Black families in therapy: A multisystems approach.* New York: Guilford Press.

Byers, D. L., Hilgenberg, C., & Rhodes, D. M. (1999). Telemedicine for patient education. *The American Journal of Distance Learning, 13,* 52–61.

Byrd, W. M., & Clayton, L. A. (2000). *An American health dilemma: A medical history of African-Americans and the problems of race beginnings to 1900.* New York: Routledge.

Byrd, W. M., & Clayton, L. A. (2002). *An American health dilemma: A medical history of African-Americans and the problems of race, medicine and health care in the United States, 1900–2000.* New York: Routledge.

Cain, J. M. (2001). Panel 1: Framing issues in rural women's health issues, Speaker 1. *Women's Health Issues, 11,* 17–21.

Campinha-Bacote, J. (1995). The quest for cultural competence in nursing care. *Nursing Forum, 30,* 136–143.

Campinha-Bacote, J. (1999). A model and instrument for addressing cultural competence in health care. *Journal of Nursing Education, 38,* 203–206.

Carrasquillo, O., Orav, E. J., Brennan, T. A., & Burstin, H. R. (1999). Impact of language barriers on patient satisfaction in an emergency department. *Journal of General Internal Medicine, 14,* 8287.

Cooper-Patrick, L., Gallo, J. J., Gonzales, J. J., Vu, H. T., Powe, N. R., Nelson, C., et al. (1999). Race, gender, and partnership in patient-physician relationship. *Journal of the American Medical Association, 282,* 583–589.

Cross, T., Bazron, B., Dennis, K., & Isaacs, M. (1989). *Towards a culturally competent system of care, Vol. 1. A monograph on effective services for minority children who are seriously emotionally disturbed.* Washington, DC: Georgetown University Child Development Center, National Technical Assistant Center for Children's Mental Health.

Dean, R. A. (2003). Native American humor: Implications for transcultural care. *Journal of Transcultural Nursing, 14,* 62–65.

Dreher, M., & Macnaughton, N. (2002). Cultural competence in nursing: Foundation or fallacy. *Nursing Outlook, 50,* 181–186.

Epstein, A. M. (1999). Quality of care by race and gender for congestive heart failure and pneumonia. *Medical Care, 37,* 1288–1294.

Fernandez, A., Schillinger, D., Grumbach, K., Rosenthal, A., Stewart, A. L., Wang, F., et al. (2004). Physician language ability and cultural competence: An exploratory study of communication with Spanish-speaking patients. *Journal of General Medicine, 19,* 167–174.

Foy, C. G., Penninx, B. W. H., Shumaker, S. A., Messier, S. P., & Pahor, M. (2005). Long-term exercise therapy resolves ethnic differences in baseline health status in older adults with knee osteoarthritis. *Journal of the American Geriatrics Society, 53,* 1469–1475.

Gamble, V. N. (1997). Under the shadow of Tuskegee: African-Americans and health care. *American Journal of Public Health, 87,* 1773–1778.

Gardner, J. (2005). Barriers to influencing the success of racial and ethnic minority students in nursing programs. *Journal of Transcultural Nursing, 16,* 155–162.

Giger, J. N., & Davidhizar, R. E. (2004). Transcultural nursing: Assessment and intervention (4th ed.). St Louis, MO: CV Mosby.

Gurwitz, J. H., Goldberg, R. J., Malmgren, J. A., Barron, H. V., Tiefenbrunn, A. J., Frederick, P. D., et al. (2002). Hospital transfer of patients with acute myocardial infarction: The effects of age, race and insurance type. *American Journal of Medicine, 112,* 528–534.

Hall, E. T. (1966). *The hidden dimension.* Garden City, NJ: Doubleday.

Hall, E. T. (1989). *Beyond culture.* New York: Doubleday.

Helman, C. G. (1990). *Culture, health, and illness* (2nd ed.). London: Butterworth.

Hilgenberg, C., & Schlickau, J. (2002). Building transcultural knowledge through intercollegiate collaboration. *Journal of Transcultural Nursing, 13,* 241–247.

Hobbs, F., & Stoops, N. (2002). *Demographic trends in the 20th century. Census 2000 special reports.* Retrieved January 19, 2006, from http://www.census.gov/prod/2002/pubs/cenr-4pdf

Institute of Medicine. (2001). *Crossing the quality chasm. A new health system for the 21st century.* Washington, DC: National Academy Press.

Institute of Medicine. (2003). *Unequal treatment: Confronting racial and ethnic disparities in health care.* Washington, DC: National Academy Press.

Jerant, A. F., Franks, P., Jackson, J. E., & Doescher, M. P. (2004). Age-related disparities in cancer screening: Analysis of 2001 Behavioral Risk Factor Surveillance System data. *Annals of Family Medicine, 2,* 481–487.

Kaplan, S. H., Gandek, B., Greenfield, S., Rogers, W., & Ware, J. E. (1995). Patient and visit characteristics related to physicians' participatory decision-making style. Results from the Medical Outcomes Study. *Medical Care, 33,* 1176–1187.

Krippner, S., & Welch, P. (1992). *Spiritual dimensions of healing.* New York: Irvington.

Laine, C., & Davidoff, F. (1996). Patient-centered medicine: A professional evolution. *Journal of the American Medical Association, 275,* 152–156.

Lazare, A., Putnam, S. M., & Lipkin, M., Jr. (1995). Three functions of the medical interview. In M. Liplin, S. Putnam, & A. Lazare (Eds.), *The Medical Interview: Clinical Care, Education and Research* (pp. 3–19). New York: Springer-Verlag.

LeClaire, M. M., Oaks, J. M., & Weinart, C. R. (2005). Communication of prognostic information for critically ill patients. *Chest, 128,* 1728–1735.

Leighton, K. (2005). Transcultural nursing: The relationship between individualistic ideology and individualized mental health care. *Journal of Psychiatric and Mental Health Nursing, 12,* 85–94.

Leininger, M. M. (1985). Transcultural diversity and universality: A theory of nursing. *Nursing and Health Care, 6,* 208–212.

Leininger, M. M. (1991). The theory of culture care diversity and universality. In M. Leininger (ed.), *Culture Care Diversity and Universality: A Theory of Nursing* (pp. 5–68). New York: National League for Nursing Press.

Leininger, M. M. (1995). Transcultural nursing. Development, focus, importance, and historical development. In M. Leininger (Ed.), *Transcultural Nursing: Concepts, Theories, Research, & Practices* (2nd ed., pp. 3–57; 115). New York: McGraw-Hill.

Leininger, M. M. (1996). Culture care theory, research and practice. *Nursing Science Quarterly, 9,* 71–78.

Leininger, M. M. (1998). What is transcultural nursing? Retrieved September 17, 2005, from http://www.tcns.org

Leininger, M. M. (2006). Culture care assessment for congruent competency practices. In M. M. Leininger & M. R. McFarland (Eds.), *Culture care diversity and universality: A worldview nursing theory* (2nd edition). Sudbury, MA: Jones and Bartlett Publishers.

Lieu, T. A., Lozano, P., Finkelstein, J. A., Chi, F. W., Jensvold, N. G., Capra, A. M., et al. (2002). Racial/ethnic variation in asthma status and management practices among children in managed care. *Pediatrics, 109,* 857–865.

Lincoln, K. (1993). *Indian humor: Bicultural play in Native America.* New York: Oxford University Press.

Lockhart, J. S., & Resnick, L. K. (1997). Teaching cultural competence: The value of experiential learning and community resources. *Nurse Educator, 22,* 27–31.

Majeed, F. A., & Cook, D. G. (1996). Age and sex differences in the management of ischemic heart disease. *Public Health, 110,* 7–12.

Malat, J. (2001). Social distance and patients' ratings of healthcare providers. *Journal of Health and Social Behaviors, 42,* 360–372.

Maples, M. F., Dupey, P., Torres-Rivera, E., Phan, L. T., Vereen, L., & Garrett, M. T. (2001). Ethnic diversity and the use of humor in counseling: Appropriate or inappropriate? *Journal of Counseling and Development, 79,* 53–60.

Mayberry, R. M., Mili, F., & Ofili, E. (2000). Racial and ethnic differences in access to medical care. *Medical Care Research Review, 57*(Suppl. 1), 108–145.

Mullins, C. D., Blatt, L., Gbarayor, C. M., Yang, H. W., & Baquet, C. (2005). Health disparities: A barrier to high-quality care. *American Journal of Health Systems Pharmacology, 62,* 1873–1882.

Murphy, V. H., Krumholz, H. M., & Gross, C. P. (2004). Participation in cancer clinical trials: Race, sex, and age-based disparities. *Journal of the American Medical Association, 291,* 2720–2726.

Nilsen, A. P., & Nilsen, D. L. F. (2000). *Encyclopedia of 20th-century American humor.* Phoenix, AZ: Oryx Press.

Núñez, A. E. (2000). Transforming cultural competence into cross-cultural efficacy in women's health education. *Academic Medicine, 75,* 1071–1080.

O'Malley, A. S., & Forrest, C. B. (2002). The mismatch between urban women's preferences for and experiences in primary care. *Women's Health Issues, 12,* 191–203.

Ory, M., Kinney Hoffman, M., Hawkins, M., Sanner, B., & Mockenhaupt, R. (2003). Challenging age stereotypes: Strategies for creating a more active society. *American Journal of Preventive Medicine, 25,* 164–171.

Padilla, R., Gomez, V., Biggerstaff, S. L., & Mehler, P. S. (2001). Use of *curanderismo* in a public health care system. *Archives of General Psychiatry, 161,* 1336–1340.

Paasche-Orlow, M (2004). The ethics of cultural competence. *Academic Medicine, 79,* 44–48.

Persell, S. D., & Baker, D. W. (2004). Aspirin use among adults with diabetes: Recent trends and emerging sex disparities. *Archives of Internal Medicine, 164,* 2492–2499.

Povlsen, L., Olsen, B., & Ladelund, S. (2005). Diabetes in children and adolescents from ethnic minorities: Barriers to education, treatment and good metabolic control. *Journal of Advanced Nursing, 50,* 576–582.

Purnell, L. (2000). A description of the Purnell model for cultural competence. *Journal of Transcultural Nursing, 11,* 40–46.

Purnell, L. D., & Paulanka, B. J. (2003). *Transcultural health care: The culturally-competent approach* (2nd ed.). Philadelphia: F. A. Davis.

Roberts, S. J. (2004). Empowering older women: Strategies to enhance their health and health care. *Journal of Obstetrics and Neonatal Nursing, 33,* 664–670

Roter, D. L., Hall, J. A., & Aoki, Y. (2002). Physician gender effects in medical communication: A meta-analytic review. *Journal of the American Medical Association, 288,* 756–764.

Satir, V. (1967). *Conjoint family therapy* (rev ed.). Palo Alto, CA: Science and Behavior Books.

Schulman, K. A., Berlin, J. A., Harless, W., Kerner, J. F., Sistrunk, S., Gersh, B. J., et al. (1999). The effect of race and sex on physicians' recommendations for cardiac catherization. *New England Journal of Medicine, 340,* 618–626.

Smedley, B. D., Stith, A. Y., & Nelson, A. R. (2003). *Unequal treatment: Confronting racial and ethnical disparities in health care.* Washington, DC: National Academies Press.

Stewart, B. (1995). Cultural considerations. In D. Antai-Otong (Ed.), *Psychiatric Nursing* (pp. 47–64). Philadelphia: W. B. Saunders.

Stewart, M., Brown, J. B., Boon, H., Galajda, J., Meredith, L., & Sangster, M. (1999). Evidence on patient-doctor communication. *Cancer Prevention Control, 3,* 25–30.

Street, R. L. Jr., Gordon, H. S., Ward, M. M., Krupat, E., & Kravitz, R. L. (2005). Patient participation in medical consultations: Why some patients are more involved than others. *Medical Care, 43,* 960–969.

Trossman, S. (1998). Diversity: A continuing challenge. *American Nurse, 30,* 24–25.

U.S. Census Bureau.(2000b). U.S. census 2000. Retrieved September 17, 2005, from http://www.census.gov; retrieved January 19, 2006, from http://www.census.gov/prod/2002/pubs/cenr-4pdf

U.S. Department of Health and Human Services. (2000). *Healthy people 2010: Understanding and improving health* (2nd ed.). Washington, DC: U.S. Government Printing Office.

U.S. Department of Health and Human Services. (2001). *The registered nurse population. National sample survey of registered nurses.* Washington, DC: Health Resources and Services Resources.

van den Brink-Muinen, A., Bensing, J. M., & Kerssens, J. J. (1998). Gender and communication style in general practice: Differences between women's health care and regular health care. *Medical Care, 36,* 100–106.

Vivian, C., & Dundes, L. (2004). The crossroads of culture and health among the Roma (Gypsies). *Image: Journal of Nursing Scholarship, 36,* 86–91.

Weisman, C. S., Rich, D. E., Rogers, J., Crawford, K. G., Grayson, C. E., & Henderson, T. J. (2000). Gender and patient satisfaction with primary care: Tuning in to women in quality measurement. *Journal of Women's Health Gender Based Medicine, 9,* 657–665.

Warren, B. J. (2003). Culture and ethnic considerations. In D. Antai-Otong (Ed.), *Psychiatric Nursing: Biological and Behavioral Concepts* (pp. 151–165). Clifton Parks, New York: Thomson Delmar Learning.

Welch, L. C., Teno, J. M., & Mor, V. (2005). End-of-life in black and white: Race matters for medical care of dying patients and their families. *Journal of the American Geriatrics Society, 53,* 1145–1153.

Zielke-Nadkarni, A. (2003). The meaning of family: Lived experiences of Turkish women immigrants in Germany. *Nursing Science Quarterly, 16,* 169–173.

SELECTED WEB SITES

Administration on Aging Resources for Minorities and Diverse Populations: http://www.aoa.gov/prof/adddiv/resources/ adddiv.html

American Translators Association: http://www.atanet.org

EthnoMed—Ethnic medicine information from Harborview Medical Center: http://www.ethnomed.org

Federal Interagency Forum on Age-Related Statistics, Older Americans 2004—Key Indicators of Well-Being: http://www.agingstats.gov

Georgetown Center for Child and Human Development, National Center for Cultural Competence—Cultural Competence Health Practitioner Assess-

ment: http://www4.georgetown.edu/uis/keybridge/keyform/form.
cfm?formID=277

Georgetown Center for Child and Human Development, National Center
for Cultural Competence—Curricula Enhancement Module Series:
http://www.nccccurricula.info

Georgetown Center for Child and Human Development, National Center
for Cultural Competence—Self-Assessment: An Essential Component of
Cultural Competence: http://gucchd.georgetown.edu/nccc/orgselfassess.
html#benefits

U.S. Department of Health and Human Services, Office of Minority
Health—Assuring Cultural Competence in Health Care: Recommendations
for National Standards and an Outcomes-Focused Research Agenda:
http://www.omhrc.gov/clas

U.S. Department of Health and Human Services, Office of Minority
Health—A Practical Guide for Implementing the Recommended National
Standards of Culturally and Linguistically Appropriate Services in Health
Care: http://www.omhrc.gov/clas/guide2a.asp

Chapter Five

Professional Development: Leading Through Effective Communication

---

LEARNING OBJECTIVES

Upon completion of this chapter, the reader should be able to:

1. Compare assertive, passive, and aggressive communication

2. Discuss key concepts of negotiation and conflict resolution

3. Describe emotional intelligence within the context of health care teams

4. Analyze various stages of group formation

5. Develop a self-renewal plan for personal development

6. Describe major components of successful public speaking

KEY TERMS

Assertiveness—The ability to express feelings, thoughts, beliefs, and rights openly, genuinely, appropriately, and respectfully without infringing on the rights of others.

Autonomy—Independence or freedom in making health care decisions within the scope of nursing practice.

Emotional intelligence—The ability to manage one's personal emotions while empathizing with and responding appropriately to others.

Empowerment—The autonomy and responsibility to make decisions and implement appropriate interventions or actions.

Evidence-based decision making—Making nursing decisions based on research or available proven scientific knowledge associated with quality health care.

Negotiation—A shared decision-making process during which two or more parties try to reach an agreement or resolve a conflict.

Personal mastery—Balancing personal life and health, career development, and lifelong learning.

Self-renewal—Personal health activities and behaviors that promote physical, mental, psychological, emotional, and spiritual well-being.

Team building—A process during which communication and leadership skills are used to work effectively with others toward common goals, reach consensus, and implement evidence-based care.

INTRODUCTION

Today's health care arena presents enormous challenges and responsibilities to nurses as they seek to actualize personal and professional goals. Mounting evidence indicates the provision of quality health care parallels a nurse's professional progress. **Personal mastery** is a core element of professional development and personal well-being through self-renewal. **Self-renewal** requires engaging in activities that promote physical, emotional, spiritual, psychosocial, and mental health (Antai-Otong, 2001). Through personal mastery the nurse becomes a visionary, a client advocate, a risk taker, and a lifelong learner. Personal mastery facilitates interpersonal effectiveness and the adaptability to work with clients and others to address vast health care issues.

High levels of motivation for professional performance and development strengthen nurses' critical thinking skills and increase confidence and empowerment to manage complex health care problems and ensure cost-effective and quality care across the health care continuum. **Empowerment** refers to the **autonomy** and responsibility to make decisions and implement appropriate interventions or actions. The ability to feel empowered and autonomous is based on personal values, self-worth, beliefs, integrity, and expertise (Kuokkanen, Leino-Kilpi, & Katajisto, 2003). Empowerment is essential to achieving high self-esteem and **assertiveness**. Through personal empowerment the nurse uses interventions that ensure clients and families are active participants in their care and in informed decision making. Because nurses, who are predominantly women, often feel disempowered, many have limited success in gaining control over their work environment, partly because of personal devaluation and failure to support each other (Daiski, 2004; MacPhee & Scott, 2002). Socialization factors contribute to these perceptions and, unless they are changed, power will continue to elude the nurse at all levels within the organization. Drastic changes are needed to address these issues. Change must begin with students, novices, and experienced nurses valuing themselves, establishing interpersonal relationships within and outside their profession, and becoming active participants in health care decision-making processes. They also must recognize the vast contributions they make in health care organizations and their impact on clinical outcomes (Daiski, 2004). (See Research Study 5-1 on pages 232–233 for findings that link key organizational attributes with advances in professional development.)

During a time of great change in methods of health care delivery, with a greater focus on cost-effectiveness, efficiency, and evidence-based care, nurses must continuously prepare to work with others to advance the needs of the client. Fortunately, these issues also resonate among health care leaders and organizations, many of whom are redesigning health care systems to shore up resources, provide **client-centered nursing care**, and implement evidence-based care across the health care continuum.

The Institute of Medicine (IOM) publication *Crossing the Quality Chasm* (2001) and its previous publication, *To Err Is Human: Building a Safer Health System,* have revolutionized health care. The IOM determined a need for basic changes in health care delivery systems. Primary emphasis was placed on the need to transform or redesign health care through integration of evidence-based processes and technologies, chronic disease management, and holistic care, and implementation by interdisciplinary teams. Six recommendations evolved from the committee:

- *Safe*—Reduce risk and avoid injury.
- *Effective*—Provide scientifically based care.
- *Client-centered*—Show respect for client preferences, lifestyles, choices, expressed needs, and values.
- *Timely*—Reduce wait times and increase access to care.
- *Efficient*—Avoid waste.
- *Equitable*—Ensure care to all populations (e.g., gender, ethnicity, culture), regardless of location and socioeconomic status. (IOM, 2001)

Recommendations from the IOM to redesign health care systems represent a paradigm shift toward chronic disease management versus care of acute episodic conditions and a community-based versus inpatient care model. A need for efficient resource allocation, increased chronic disease management, and a focus on client-centered care requires health care that optimizes resources and staff. Interdisciplinary teams, collaboration, and effective communication among nurses, clients, families, and health care professionals offer such solutions. This paradigm shift is pivotal in the integration of technologies and the provision of quality and client-centered nursing care. As the client accesses care and navigates the health care continuum their personal health data must accompany them to ensure a seamless plan of care. Well-crafted, evidence-based care processes, supported by electronic information technologies and decision support systems, provide the most efficient processes with which to attain quality and positive clinical outcomes (IOM, 2001).

New rules or recommendations proposed by the IOM report also have impacted the role, self-image, and health processes of nurses and health care professionals. Transitions in health care delivery call for nurses and other health care providers to learn new skills and interactions to relate to clients and each other. Inherent in these recommendations are increased responsibilities for nurses and other clinicians to collaborate and partner with clients and families to ensure shared decision making, self-management, and individualized and evidence-based care. Because nurses are concerned with human responses and needs across the life span, partnerships with the client, family, and other health care professionals provide a venue to address a myriad of health care issues and concerns, such as health promotion, adherence to treatment, self-care management, and willingness to embrace the client's experience (American Nurses Association [ANA], 2003).

As providers of health care and participants on interdisciplinary teams, nurses have tremendous responsibilities involving implementation of redesigned health care. Accordingly, all nurses must be prepared to communicate and lead within diverse social contexts to advance seamless health care. Cohesive interdisciplinary teams are difficult to form for a variety of reasons, including an organizational culture that impedes shared decision making or members' poor communication and conflict resolution skills. Well-designed teams operate under the assumption that each member is a valued participant in the health care decision-making process. Members are also expected to share their expertise and knowledge, collaborate, develop and implement treatments to meet complex client needs, and facilitate positive clinical outcomes (ANA, 2003; Bulger, 2000).

As health care transitions, so must nurses' roles. Today's nurses must place a greater emphasis on professional development, effective communication, team building, and leadership. Professional development and leadership skills are dynamic and ever-changing and must meet the needs of the nurse, client, family, staff, health care organization, and community. Numerous studies indicate the impact of healthy work environments and supportive leadership on the nurse's ability to succeed and develop professionally within an organization. Nurse leaders are accountable for designing and enunciating organizational values, vision, and role delineation that sanction innovative and flexible roles and create work environments that encourage success and professional development (National Institute of Standards and Technology, 2000). Healthy work environments are grounded in staff and client satisfaction, appropriate and equitable resource allocation, and professional development through open communication that increases staff morale, individual decision making, confidence, and healthy interpersonal relationships (Nolan, Lundh, & Brown, 1999).

This chapter addresses key concepts associated with advancing professional development—motivating and influencing others and creating work environments that optimize resources and the overall well-being of clients, families, staff, the health care organization and communities. As students, novices, or experienced nurses formulate their personal vision of self and others within diverse social contexts it is imperative that they become effective communicators and leaders both at the bedside and within organizational hierarchies.

WHAT CONSTITUTES AN EFFECTIVE LEADER?

Influential leadership and communication skills are essential aspects of professional development, clinical competence, job satisfaction, and continuous learning. Advancing quality health care across the health care continuum requires confidence, realistic expectations of self and others, emotional intelligence, self-esteem, and motivation to succeed. Distinct principles govern effective leadership competencies and professional development, such as motivation, emotional intelligence, self-awareness, assertiveness, and healthy interpersonal relationships. Emerging paradigm shifts and redesigned health care systems call for nurse leaders with broad clinical expertise, interpersonal and critical thinking skills, flexibility, and emotional intelligence.

Emotional intelligence is the ability to manage one's emotions to help others within the context of establishing interpersonal relationships, conveying empathy, and responding appropriately (Freshman & Rubino, 2002; Goleman, 1996, 1998). Although this concept is relatively new in nursing, its roots arise from social psychology literature. Despite its novelty in nursing, emotional intelligence has been introduced in the nursing literature (Freshman & Rubino; Herbert & Edgar, 2004; Rochester, Kilstoff, & Scott, 2005). Theoretically, emotional intelligence is fundamental to self-awareness. It helps the nurse glean an understanding of personal reactions to nurse–client and other relationships and determine the critical interpersonal skills needed to respond appropriately. Debate regarding its relevance to nursing continues, but many consider it an important communication and leadership skill that helps front-line nurses work effectively with clients and the interdisciplinary team (Humphreys, Brunsen, & Davis, 2005; McQueen, 2004; Reeves, 2005; Rochester, Kilstoff, & Scott).

Goleman, Boyatzis, and McKee (2003) further refined the concept of emotional intelligence as four core domains of effective leadership:

* *Self-awareness*—Involves personal competence, integrity, and awareness of how emotions influence decision making and interpersonal relationships
* *Self-management or self-regulation*—Refers to effectively managing emotions; focusing on and using intellect and clinical judgment versus being controlled by impulses and quick, inappropriate, or "knee-jerk" decision making, which jeopardize the rights of others
* *Social awareness*—Involves how one relates to others and includes mindfulness and sensitivity to others, systems thinking, "looking at the bigger picture," and duty to clients, families, colleagues, and organization
* *Relationship management or social skills*—Refers to how one works with and collaborates with others, resolves conflicts, nurtures, and facilitates optimal function and performance in self and others

You may want to consider using emotional intelligence for personal and professional development to strengthen self-control and empathy and to enhance interpersonal relationships. Positive results of maintaining emotional intelligence include expanded self-awareness within the social context of others, increased empathy, improved interpersonal relationships, increased job satisfaction, and positive clinical outcomes. Together, self-awareness, self-management, social awareness, and relationship management offer students, novices, and experienced nurses a means to explore issues that generate strong anxiety and discomfort and their actual and potential impact on decision making and interpersonal relationships. Effective leadership requires balancing emotions and intellect through self-awareness and diverting energies constructively to ensure healthy work relationships and greater leadership effectiveness. Frequently, this balancing act is difficult because it may go unrecognized or misunderstood. Recognizing and understanding the potential positive and negative impacts of your emotional states on client care is crucial to using emotions to make sound clinical judgments, interact with others, and maintain quality interpersonal relationships. An in-depth discussion of self-awareness is provided in Chapters 1 and 2.

Professional and leadership development also require a desire to change and flexibility and adaptation to the daily hassles of work environments and interpersonal encounters. Noted national organizational consultants Bennis and Townsend (1995) submit that the following are qualities of an effective leader:

- *Keeps personal ambitions under control*—This means keeping your ego in check, recognizing the importance of open communication, and being willing to listen to, value, and appreciate others while focusing on personal goals. The antithesis of keeping your ego in check is aggressively meeting personal goals by destroying the rights of others—either through verbal abuse, personal attacks, or disrespect. By focusing solely on personal goals, the nurse fails to embrace the wisdom, knowledge, and expertise of others and eventually erodes trust and interpersonal relationships.
- *Is knowledgeable and intelligent*—Opportunities for professional involvement are vast and include participating in or leading workgroups that examine legislative and practice issues that impact nursing practice, attending and presenting at national and local conferences, and working on various professional task groups. These also provide invaluable opportunities to network with nurse leaders and explore opportunities for mentoring and preceptorship. Learning and professional development are continuous processes during which the nurse must stay abreast of legislative, practice, and research issues impacting practice.
- *Is articulate and has good communication skills*—Getting your message across to others using effective communication skills is pivotal to professional development. Whether you are doing a presentation or short discussion during an interdisciplinary team meeting or providing health

education to a client and family, you must be able to speak well and be understood. Most people feel anxious when asked to lead a meeting, do short presentations, or even provide health education, but you are not alone. Performance anxiety is common and is sometimes paralyzing to nurses. It often stems from a fear of ridicule, humiliation, or poor performance and frequently interferes with advancing personal and professional goals. (A detailed discussion of public speaking is provided later in this chapter.) Recognizing your anxiety level and underlying fears about communicating with others is crucial to resolving it. Attributes of effective communication include:

- ○ Active listening
- ○ Good eye contact (while considering cultural influences)
- ○ Open body language
- ○ Paraphrasing
- ○ Reflective listening
- ○ Appropriate distance
- ○ Congruent verbal and nonverbal body language
- ○ Normal voice tone

(An in-depth discussion of specific therapeutic communication skills is found in Chapter 2.)

- *Provides opportunities for others to succeed*—Personal value and self-worth enable the nurse to respect the rights of self and others. Because of gender issues and socialization, some nurses find it difficult to succeed and hence put up barriers that impede others from succeeding. Personal development requires a vision, believing in the right to succeed, mentoring, and accommodating an environment that encourages others to succeed. Valuing colleagues and staff means being committed to their satisfaction, success, and sense of well-being. A negative perception of clients or outcomes associated with specific treatments is communicated through both verbal and nonverbal communication.

Every opportunity must be afforded for others to succeed. People tend to treat others the way they feel about themselves. Positive self-perception and self-confidence are contagious. By creating a supportive climate and environment of open communication people develop and grow from others' successes. Inconsistent findings support this premise, but most indicate supportive work environments may mitigate workplace stress and burnout and improve performance and job satisfaction (AbuAlRub, 2004;

MacPhee & Scott, 2002; Wade, 2004). (See Research Study 5-2 on pages 233–234 for a further discussion of the importance of supportive relationships among nurses.)

Supportive relationships are vital to healthy work relationships. This tenet reflects the ANA's (2004) *Nursing: Scope and Standards of Practice* publication, which states "the registered nurse interacts and contributes to the professional development of peers and colleagues" (p. 37). Nurse leaders must create supportive work environments for frontline nurses and foster self-confidence and assertiveness (Kane & Thomas, 2000) through mentoring and preceptorship during various stages in the nurse's career (Mills, Francis, & Bonner, 2005).

Mentoring affords unique opportunities to succeed. It has implications for role socialization and development and is equally important for health outcomes. It is an important aspect of professional development and role development for novice and experienced nurses. Personal development necessitates seeking opportunities to form these relationships, and nurse leadership must sanction these initiatives and encourage mentoring and preceptorship. Mentoring is mutually beneficial to both the mentor and mentee, with advantages such as strengthening communication and leadership skills and helping the mentee traverse care across the health continuum and understand intricate organizational hierarchies that impact nursing practice.

Nurse leaders have a responsibility to nurture novice and experienced nurses and address recruitment and retention issues by creating avenues for lifelong career and professional development. This requires open communication among nurses, clients, clinicians, and stakeholders. Naturally, each nurse is responsible for his or her own professional development; however, unless the organization embraces this concept, nurses will continue to struggle to achieve personal and professional goals and will become increasingly apathetic and dissatisfied. Open communication galvanizes trust, increases altruism, improves productivity, mitigates interpersonal conflict, and promotes job satisfaction and staff morale. Nurse job satisfaction has been correlated with perceived accomplishments, autonomy, appreciation, and inherent enthusiasm in the nurse's work environment (Healy & McKay, 2000).

- *Uses factual and earnest decision making*—A nonjudgmental attitude and willingness to value and embrace others' ideas and beliefs increases objectivity and fairness and reduces biases generated by differences between self and others. Self-awareness is an integral part of earnest decision making.

As mentioned in previous chapters, nurses must understand their own beliefs, values, and perceptions of health and illness and how subjectivity impacts interactions with and perception of others. Culture, ethnicity, socioeconomic status, education level, and other factors play pivotal roles in perceptions and beliefs about self and others. Left unchecked, subjectivity contributes to mistrust, inaccurate interpretation of signs and symptoms, misdiagnosis, inappropriate goal setting, and, subsequently, inept interventions, which produce poor clinical outcomes.

- *Finds humor even when things go wrong*—Effective leadership requires an ability to celebrate successes and grow from adversities and failures. Supportive environments, empathy, and acceptance of differences is the basis of growing from failures and moving towards success. Seeing the humorous side of failures or negative situations requires confidence and high self-esteem. A positive attitude enables the nurse to reevaluate what went wrong and generate ideas to validate goals that are realistic, measurable, and appropriate. A failure to view these situations as growth enhancing prevents resolution and jeopardizes professional and personal development. It is imperative to remember that a failure just means starting over again; the advantage of this premise is that it puts the event in perspective and allows the nurse to regroup, learn from the experience, and frame it positively rather negatively.

- *Has integrity and wisdom*—Integrity infers honesty and adherence to moral and ethical principles. Wisdom refers to the quality of scholarly knowledge or learning and/or insight. Lifelong experiences involving critical thinking skills, growth from failures, and successes are the cornerstone of wisdom and integrity. Integrity and wisdom are the basis of effective and persuasive leadership. They must be used to create and guide health care environments that instill sound clinical decision making and ethical principles. Integrity and wisdom must be communicated behaviors demonstrated by nurse leadership and the organization's behavior and culture. Through professional activities and practice, students and nurses glean the basis of the organization's vision, mission, and values concerning health care. Nurse leaders are in key positions to instill these principles through career and professional development. Educational opportunities as well as financial support to attend conferences and maintain national certification are examples of organizational support for career development. (Antai-Otong, 1999)

An organizational culture in which nurses are valued, collaborative relationships are endorsed, quality outcomes are demonstrated, and high-quality physicians and specialists are attracted can receive a *magnet designation*. The Magnet Recognition Program was developed by the American Nurses Credentialing Center (ANCC), an ancillary of the American Nurses Association, during the 1980s and early 1990s, and recognizes health care systems for excellence in nursing services (ANCC, 2005). Magnet designation indicates quality and excellence in nursing service and exemplifies professionalism (ANCC). Researchers submit that magnet cultures consistently surpass their competitors in recruiting and retaining nurses (Aiken, Clarke, Sloan, Sochalski, & Silber, 2002). Although most health care systems have not attained magnet recognition, nurse leaders must seek to create environments that recognize the unique contributions of nurses, provide opportunities for professional development, and reinforce positive collaborative relationships. Browse the ANCC Web site for criteria to attain the magnet designation (http://www.nursingworld.org/ancc/magnet/consumer/whatis4.html).

Major challenges of creating these environments include a lack of confidence, poor leadership, and weak communication skills in nurses who are in a position to create healthy work cultures; they also may be unwilling to take risks for fear of reprisal. Historically, nurse leaders have failed to create supportive work relationships and an environment conducive to professional development. As a result there is a lack of unity and solidarity among nurses that continues to dilute their power within the organization and bedside, and to suppress their creativity (Daiski, 2004). More significantly, without supportive work environments and relationships that strengthen leadership and communication skills, nurses will continue to falter in their quest for power and understanding of systems thinking.

SYSTEMS THINKING

The concept of systems thinking must be an integral part of professional nursing. It generates knowledge of organizational hierarchies that impact health care and decision making. It is imperative for all nurses to understand organizational hierarchies to prepare for special assignment on different units or clinic areas. This familiarizes the nurse with key decision makers and lines of communication within the organization and strengthens system thinking.

Frontline or bedside nurses must develop communication and interpersonal skills that enable them to view their workplace and health care from the "big picture perspective" and work within various systems in a changing health care arena. Emphasis on strong collaborative relationships with clients, staff, and stakeholders is critical to this process. A greater focus on efficiency, appropriate resource allocation, and individualized care involves enhancing mutual interests and emphasizing relatedness, clinical outcomes, and vertical orientation (Porter-O'Grady & Malloch, 2003). By using systems thinking the nurse is able to see his or her organization as a whole system and distinguish the characteristics of various hierarchies and their contributions to the entire organization.

Modern health care requires leaders on the frontline and in the boardroom to gain and use control and power effectively to advance quality health care and create environments that expect open communication and engender trust, a sense of well-being, and support for staff development and restoration of health. Boundaries among staff and clients must be fluid enough to encourage integration of new information, technologies, and research as a basis of quality health outcomes. Communication is critical to this process and requires clear and articulate interpersonal skills, confidence, and assertiveness. The next section focuses on assertiveness as a core quality of personal development and collaboration, and a necessary skill to navigate complex organizational hierarchies and advance holistic nursing care across the health care continuum.

PROFESSIONAL ASSERTIVENESS

As discussed in Chapter 2, assertive nurses have the confidence in their judgment and the high self-esteem needed to openly express their thoughts, feelings, and beliefs in a genuine, appropriate, and respectful manner. Assuring the rights of self and others is the core of assertiveness. Assertive communication also means using congruent verbal and nonverbal communication, through which the nurse clearly describes the concern or problem from a personal perspective, expresses feelings in a nonthreatening manner, and lists or specifies desirable behaviors and choices for him- or herself and others. The ultimate goal of assertiveness is to meet one's needs and ensure personal rights while assuring others' rights (Bower & Bower, 1976). Assertiveness requires courage, personal respect, common sense, honesty, and risk taking (see Table 5-1). This skill is often a blend of innate attributes and learned experiences gleaned through positive early interactions with parents or caregivers and professional opportunities that strengthen mindfulness, self-assuredness, and achievement. Organizational leadership and work environments must create vast opportunities for the nurse to develop assertive communication skills.

Table 5-1 Essential Characteristics of Professional Assertiveness

Characteristics	Behaviors
Self-assuredness	Use "I" or "me" statements.
Confidence	Use good eye contact.
Risk taking	Attempt to resolve the problem at the
Willingness to "think outside the box"	lowest level to facilitate healthy resolution
Respect for self and others	and maintain trust.
Honesty and sincerity	
Empathy	
Self-control	
Emotional intelligence	
Open and clear communication skills	

In the past nurses were discouraged from being assertive and rewarded for being passive—these behaviors reflected societal expectations. Now, however, unless the nurse communicates assertively, she or he will remain outside of important relationships responsible for clinical decision making and implementation of health care. Even when nurses are assertive, a prevailing fear of retribution and negative reactions from others discourages this behavior. Socialization pressures associated with being female and putting others' needs ahead of their own helped to create the negative image of assertive women. In modern health care environments, assertiveness is no longer a luxury, but a necessity. Students, novices, and experienced nurses must be prepared to be assertive and communicate effectively to advance personal developmental goals and establish collaborative relationships with their colleagues and clients to ensure quality clinical outcomes. A failure to develop and use these skills lowers self-esteem, creates uncertainty, and engenders anger, burnout, oppression, ineffectual work relationships, and negative clinical outcomes (Freeman & Adams, 1999). Negative clinical outcomes often stem from a lack of the communication and leadership skills necessary to collaborate with clients, colleagues, and stakeholders and participate in shared decision making. Table 5-2 lists some helpful assertive communication patterns.

SHARED DECISION MAKING

A growing body of research shows a strong link between shared decision making with clients and improved positive clinical outcomes (Beach et al., 2005; Edwards et al., 2004). According to the IOM (2001), the freedom to

Table 5-2 Specific Assertive Communication Patterns

Behavior	Example
Clearly state your concerns.	"I am very upset . . .
Describe the behavior.	. . . because you raised your voice in the staff meeting this morning."
Discuss the consequences of the other's behaviors.	"When you raised your voice I felt fearful and embarrassed."
Suggest ways to avoid the behavior in the future.	"In the future, when you speak to me I would appreciate you lowering your voice and speaking to me one on one rather than yelling in a group."

participate in shared decision making is a *fundamental* value and right of every client in contemporary health care systems. Shared decision making must parallel client preferences, needs, lifestyles, and wishes and reflect evidence-based practice. This principle suggests that *"client values drive variability"* (IOM, 2001, p. 71) in health care decisions. Culture, gender, generation, and ethnicity must govern the treatment of each client (Carrillo, Green, & Betancourt, 1999; Smith, 1998). Health education is an integral component of shared decision making.

Health education provides the information necessary to make informed decisions unique to personal needs, cultures, and preferences. Most clients want to understand treatment choices and participate in decision making consistent with their culture, ethnicity, and gender needs, wishes, and decisions (Harrison, 2000). Health education lies within the domain of nursing and is based on individual client needs, preferences, values, beliefs, and health practices. Nurse–client relationships provide excellent forums for engaging clients and their families in the shared decision-making process based on clinical choices to mitigate symptoms and achieve optimal health outcomes. To achieve optimal health outcomes the nurse must be able to collaborate with clients and families with various illnesses so that they commit to and adhere to treatment recommendations. Several approaches enhance this process:

- *Ask open-ended questions*—"How have you managed these symptoms in the past?" versus "Have you been treated for these symptoms before?"
- *Give clear directions*—"Mr. Jones, this medication needs to be taken at the same time every morning to establish a regular schedule" versus "Take this medication every day."
- *Avoid interruptions*—"Please finish your question" versus "Just a minute, I think you need to do. . . ."

- *Elicit input from the client and involve him or her in the decision-making process*—"Mrs. Murphy, here is a list of things you can do to improve sleep. Let me know which one you prefer" versus "Mrs. Murphy, do not drink tea before going to bed."

Enlisting the client and family in the decision-making process facilitates mutual definition of problems; enhances treatment planning, management strategies, and self-management skills, especially for chronic disease; and encourages independence. Research indicates that this approach increases the quality of clients' health care, emotional health, symptom relief, and autonomy and accountability for specific aspects of their care, and achieves adherence to treatment (Beach et al., 2005; Clark et al., 2000; Edwards et al., 2004; Lorig et al., 2001).

Whereas most clients enjoy the autonomy and independence of shared decision making, some clients prefer to have other people make their health care decisions for them. Research also indicates that some clients relinquish decision making to their physicians; this often depends on the nature of the decision, particularly for older adults, and the seriousness of the illness (Arora & McHorney, 2000; Mansell, Poses, Kazis, & Duefield, 2000; Stiggelbout & Kiebert, 1997). Although some clients may prefer to delegate decision making to the nurse, physician, and health care team, they must be afforded opportunities to exercise their right to participate in the process and make informed decisions.

Creating environments that facilitate client-centered health care and active participation in decision making may generate personal reflection regarding one's own culture, decisions, and health practices. Self-awareness of the impact of these issues provides a forum for the nurse to explore personal reactions, biases, and variables that may impede effective nurse–client interactions. (See Georgetown University's Cultural Competence Self-Assessment under Selected Web Sites at the end of this chapter.)

Cultural and Ethnic Influences on Shared Decision Making

The U.S. population is becoming increasingly more culturally diverse. This growing diversity requires a greater emphasis on addressing the needs of individuals from a variety of cultural backgrounds. Issues such as gender, poverty, language spoken, place of birth, previous negative experiences with health care providers, degree of integration within the ethnic or cultural community, socioeconomic status, biological factors, and educational preparation impact individual preferences and needs (Crawley, Marshall, & Koenig, 2001; Veatch, 2000).

Culture, ethnicity, and religious and spiritual beliefs shape client choices and health practices; interpersonal relationships; roles within a social context; perceptions of health, suffering, and dying; expectations of care; treatment decisions; and various aspects of care. Nurses and other clinicians face the challenge of caring for clients from diverse cultures who use a variety of languages, have different levels of acculturation, and have unique ways of grasping the meaning of health and illness. Nurses must use *every* nurse–client encounter to understand each client's unique experiences. Learning about the uniqueness and richness of culture evolves through nurse–client relationships (Campinha-Bacote, 1999).

Most people have varied cultural and ethnic backgrounds that extend beyond race, ethnicity, and place of origin (Betancourt, 2004). Accordingly, effective nurse leaders must also recognize how their own culture shapes and frames other people's perceptions, communication patterns, and health care practices. As frontline leaders, nurses must assess the cultural and spiritual needs of their clients across the health care continuum to ensure holistic nursing care and facilitate an optimal level of functioning.

A culturally sensitive assessment is grounded in the nurse's knowledge of a client's lifestyle, wishes, decisions, and unique physical, biological, and psychological distinctions that govern the nurse's ability to perform a physical evaluation (Purnell, 2002; Purnell & Paulanka, 2003). (See Chapter 4 for a discussion of the cultural aspects of communication.) The client's cultural, religious, and spiritual beliefs must be assessed and integrated in the shared decision-making process.

Cultural competence or sensitivity requires self-awareness of personal beliefs and values and their actual or potential impact on how the nurse interacts with the client, families, and colleagues. A greater concern is how culture and ethnicity influence the way the nurse communicates information about the client and family to staff and members of the interdisciplinary team. Nurses must explore their attitudes about certain ethnic or cultural groups and recognize verbal and nonverbal cues that convey intolerance, a lack of sensitivity, and prejudices. A failure to recognize one's personal biases and their influence on nurse–client or nurse–family encounters in shared decision making can have detrimental effects on the nurse–client/ nurse–family relationship and clinical outcomes. Evidence of biases and prejudice toward specific populations include comments such as:

- Why bother? He's not going to understand anyway.
- They never follow instructions. That's why he's back in the hospital again.
- Those people never try.

- Why don't they learn to speak our language?
- Why does her husband continuously answer questions for her?
- Her mother and father are too controlling.

When these types of questions or comments occur, what is your response? Do you walk away or ignore them? Do you become angry and aggressive, and point out how wrong they are? How often do nurses take these opportunities to educate themselves and others about cultural competence? Nurse leaders both at the frontline and in the boardroom must address these issues as real and explore avenues to education all staff to ensure cultural competence and sensitivity. Essential principles of cultural competence include:

- Value and recognition of the significance of culture in individual's lives
- High regard for cultural diversity
- Accepting and valuing differences
- Mitigating negative or adverse consequences of cultural differences
- Promoting these principles by learning about culture, embracing pluralism, and anticipating unique needs based on client choices, health practices, beliefs, and values (Paasche-Orlow, 2004)

Acknowledging the impact of culture on health practices, beliefs and values, and responses to illness and health helps the nurse integrate client needs into practice and facilitates factual data collection and analysis and the implementation of appropriate and individualized care. A more important issue is how self-awareness or red flags that guide our communication and relational processes and influences how we listen to and understand our clients. Typically red flags are depicted as unfounded anger or anxiety, discounting or minimizing the client's concerns, wishes, preferences, and complaints. A failure to respond to these red flags and acknowledge the needs of diverse cultures and ethnicities will damage the nurse–client relationship, staff morale, interpersonal relationships among staff, and clients' clinical outcomes. Cultural sensitivity and competence must be an integral part of nursing. They promote understanding of the relevance and significance of race and ethnic background on the shared decision-making process.

Inquiring about each client's health care choices, wishes, beliefs, and health practices rather than speculating allows the nurse to develop a greater understanding of the client's experience and obviates embarrassing situations. The benefits of cultural competence are enormous. It expands the quality of nurse–client relationships and increases the success rate of the encounter; research indicates cultural competence has a positive impact on treatment adherence and clinical outcomes (IOM, 2001; Scott, 1997; Stewart et al., 1999; Welch, 1998). A failure to assess and address the meaning of the client's experiences and culture often generates mistrust, nonadherence to treatment, and poor health outcomes (Antai-Otong, 2002; Stewart et al.). As brokers of quality and client-centered health care, nurses are obligated to develop and initiate processes that help clients and families navigate health care systems and gain timely access to treatment (see Table 5-3). (See Chapter 4: Cultural Aspects of Communication Partnerships.)

Shared decision making is a fundamental right of every client. Acquisition of shared decision-making skills requires motivation to learn and intentional effort. It also requires a willingness to share power and control with clients and colleagues to ensure the good of the whole organization. Nurses learn what they want to learn. Through personal development, the student, novice, and experienced nurse can acquire critical leadership skills necessary to advance equitable, quality, and client-centered nursing care and exercise-shared decision making through interpersonal relationships with clients, families, and interdisciplinary team members.

Table 5-3 Suggestions to Facilitate Culturally Sensitive Shared Decision Making

- Establish your credibility, concern, and interest.
- Create an atmosphere of mutual trust.
- Learn about the dominant culture and ethnic groups in your health care system.
- Assess how decisions are made within the client's family/culture.
- Who is the primary decision maker in the home?
- What is the client/family's spoken language?
- What language is preferred during the assessment or treatment?
- Take time to listen.
- Respect the client's role in the family.
- Recognize that a history of mistrust of clinicians impacts the client/family's ability to trust and form a meaningful relationship.
- Understand the effect of culture on verbal and nonverbal communication cues.
- Focus on individual clients rather than on the presumed cultural characteristics of various cultures and ethnic groups.
- Speak to be understood.
- Explore the meaning of the client's experience or illness.
- Ascertain the names of key family members and their role in the shared decision-making process.
- Consider using an interpreter for clients with limited English proficiency rather than using a family member as an interpreter.

CONFLICT MANAGEMENT

Conflicts are a natural part of human interactions. The quality of a person's conflict-management and problem-solving skills is grounded in early care-givers or parents who instilled confidence, self-esteem, and self-worth, as well as lifelong experiences and successes. Acknowledging the inherent nature of conflicts in all interpersonal relationships is the first step to resolving them. Nurses often find it difficult to resolve conflicts for various reasons, including gender-related socialization issues (e.g., oppression, helplessness), low self-esteem and confidence, and poor communication and conflict resolution skills. Vast changes in today's health care climate require effective navigation skills to ensure quality and safe care across the continuum. It is unacceptable to enter health care environments without the conflict management and negotiation skills necessary to navigate complex hierarchies and interact with diverse client populations. Minimizing, ignoring, or avoiding conflicts breeds mistrust, passive-aggressive and aggressive behaviors, contentious interpersonal relationships, low staff morale, and poor clinical outcomes.

Conflict refers to a mental struggle stemming from opposing demands, perspectives, or needs. Many different causes contribute to conflict, including the following:

- Status
- Gender
- Position and role
- Culture, including geographic differences
- Ethnicity
- Race
- Religion
- Education level
- Personality
- Socioeconomic status
- Stress
- Poor communication skills
- Values, beliefs, lifestyles, and decisions
- Perceptions
- Intolerance or rigid thinking
- Cognitive impairment
- Disorganized thought processes
- Sensory deficits

Effective conflict resolution requires understanding personal feelings linked to the conflict or dispute, using one's intellect to communicate rather than being controlled by emotions, focusing on the problem or behavior and not the individual, communicating assertively, and generating potential solutions or options. Assertive communication is critical to successful conflict resolution. Poor communication skills or passiveness or aggression can prove detrimental to effective conflict management and interpersonal relationships.

Review the following Critical Thinking Question and consider how you would handle this situation.

CRITICAL THINKING QUESTION

One of your nurse colleagues is upset with a physician on the interdisciplinary team; during a team meeting she is quiet, yet obviously upset. She folds her arms and avoids eye contact with team members and remains quiet throughout the morning meeting. Afterward she approaches you and asks you to talk to the physician because she is so upset she will say the wrong thing. As her colleague and a member of the interdisciplinary team, what is the best response to her request?

A. Set a time to meet with the physician because your colleague is obviously upset.

B. Listen to your colleague's concerns, but encourage her to talk to the physician one on one.

C. Let her know that you are unwilling to fight her battles and she needs to stand up for herself.

D. Ask her to discuss the matter with other members of the team for feedback.

There is no single "right" answer to this scenario. The correct answer must be based on knowledge of the nurse–physician relationship prior to today's meeting and the nature of their conflict. It is equally important to ascertain the nurse's assertiveness and conflict management skills. Often, asking others to resolve conflicts indicates a lack of these skills and the confidence to use them. Afterwards it is imperative to be supportive and empathetic, while encouraging colleagues to problem solve, use assertive communication, and successfully resolve interpersonal conflicts.

NEGOTIATION SKILLS

Negotiation is a shared decision-making process during which two or more parties try to reach an agreement or resolve a conflict. Negotiations are an integral part of most encounters; whether it entails negotiating with your 5-year-old to eat his breakfast or wash his face or convincing your spouse you really can afford a trip to Hawaii, everyone negotiates. Students, novices, and even experienced nurses perceive negotiation as an intimidating process. However, nurses negotiate daily—every time someone asks you to do something or vice versa. Daily negotiations range from talking to a salesperson about a reduced department store item to asking your client to take a shower in the evening instead of the morning. For instance, Mr. Jones has been discharged, but his wife is unable to pick him up as scheduled at 10 AM. You already have an early afternoon admission. The admission clerk calls and asks when Mr. Jones is going to leave because the new client has already arrived. Prior to the call, you have already negotiated with Mr. Jones's wife to pick him up around noon. You explore options with the clerk and the new client's physician and negotiate a time for her admission. Negotiation requires a give and take approach amenable to all parties. This scenario demonstrates how the nurse used effective communication and negotiation skills to ensure both clients' needs were met, while maintaining an amicable relationship with the admission clerk. Although this scenario seems inconsequential, it was not. A failure to negotiate with Mr. Jones, his wife, the new client, the doctor, and the clerk could have resulted in anger, client dissatisfaction, staff frustration, the unnecessary involvement of other parties, and inordinate time consumption to smooth things over.

Some organizational consultants state that everything is negotiable if you acquire the skills necessary to negotiate. Skopec and Kiely (1994) suggest six essential ingredients of successful negotiation:

- *An optimistic or positive attitude*—This sets the tone of the encounter and governs how others respond to you. This feature also impacts the emotional level of the interaction and facilitates dialogue and exchange of ideas and options. Eventually, first interactions become the cornerstone of the relationship. This was demonstrated in the scenario involving the client, his wife, and the clerk. Obviously the nurse had established a relationship with the involved parties, which facilitated the negotiation process. Optimism also enabled the nurse to depersonalize the situation and expect a positive outcome.

- *Knowledge of the negotiation process*—This process is often governed by the parties involved and what is at stake. Clearly the nurse in the scenario understood how important it was to establish relationships with the involved parties, to explore the options and interests of others, to suggest ways to resolve the situation and receive input from all parties involved in the process, and to agree on a plan of action. A working relationship with a client or colleague where trust, understanding, respect, and value already exist makes the negotiation process much easier and more efficient. In comparison, a failure to establish rapport and productive dialogue are detrimental to the negotiation process and interpersonal relationships.
- *Interpersonal skills or understanding of people*—This feature involves interpersonal skills that facilitate dialogue and open communication channels, enhance understanding of normal stress reactions, and focus on matters at hand rather than becoming defensive or personalizing the process. Stress generates strong emotions in all parties, but the nurse must role model behavior that indicates an understanding of people's uniqueness, needs, and preferences. Successful negotiation requires focusing on the real problem and maintaining a quality relationship. Open and clear communication is essential to negotiation. Sometimes it is helpful to put yourself in the other person's shoes to glean an understanding of their perceptions concerning the conflict. By understanding their side, the nurse can also consider solutions consistent with the other parties' values and beliefs. Avoid reacting to emotional outbursts and self-manage your own emotions.
- *Acquisition of the subject matter or issue*—Normally this refers to data gathering and having your facts straight when you enter negotiations. In this particular situation the nurse had most of the facts and understood the clients' and clerk's concerns, and therefore was able to effectively negotiate times for the discharge of one client and admission of the other.
- *Creativity*—Refers to a willingness to "think outside the box" or take risks to ensure a quality negotiation process. Each situation is different and requires open-mindedness. Creativity and ingenuity offer the nurse more options with which to negotiate.
- *Effective communication skills*—Obviously assertive communication is critical to successful negotiation. Without communication there is no negotiation; however, communication is often difficult during negotiations because of high emotions and sometimes an unwillingness to listen to the other person's side. Attentiveness to others directs their attention to

you. Ask questions to learn and understand the other party's perspective. Active listening is crucial during this process, which entails using congruent verbal and nonverbal communication to ensure an accurate message is conveyed and to minimize misunderstanding. Active listening also includes acknowledging feelings, paraphrasing, reflection, and using nonverbal cues (e.g., nodding head, using open body language). Acknowledging feelings or the other person's perspective does not infer agreement. Conflict resolution or negotiation is doubtful until the individual feels heard and understood. Negotiation involving shared decision making with the client and family is difficult when the nurse believes his or her way is the only way. Effective conflict resolution requires the nurse and client to accommodate and accept differences—negotiating some issues while remaining firm about other issues. This process creates an environment of mutual trust and shared decision making.

The quality of communication with clients, families, and team members is a crucial component in negotiation and team building. Throughout the negotiation process the nurse must speak to be understood and with a purpose and focus on self rather than the other party. Reconcile interests, rather than perspectives, and seek mutual interests and gains. As brokers of health care, nurses must recognize the importance of negotiation and use it to work effectively with others to advance quality health care. This leadership skill is a crucial part of team building and establishing productive interpersonal relationships.

TEAM-BUILDING SKILLS

Acquisition of **team-building** skills is critical to successful integration of various interdisciplinary approaches to treatment planning and positive clinical outcomes. Team-building skills help the nurse look beyond individual contributions and expertise and grasp the "big picture" or system thinking, and how the parts interface with the whole.

Team-building skills require value, character, integrity of self and others, clinical knowledge and expertise, connection, responsibility and service, altruism, accountability, and quality. Working with colleagues, clients, and families requires predictability, competence, and consistency. Keeping promises, demonstrating competency to lead and provide safe care, and showing up on time engender trust and security and personify integrity and character. Team members must be able to depend upon each other and expect members to use sound clinical judgment and make individual and team decisions based on evidence-based practice and expertise.

Trust, respect, and support are grounded in putting the needs of the team ahead of personal agendas or needs, acknowledging blunders, making firm clinical decisions, keeping promises, and following through on team assignments. Trust among team members evolves over time and is facilitated by effective team-building processes, quality communication structures, conflict management, problem solving, and leadership skills. Socialization requires getting beyond "me" to an "us" or "we" attitude and valuing each member's uniqueness and role on the team. Trust and quality socialization enable the nurse to express feelings and thoughts appropriately using assertive communication skills, focus on the positives and improvement issues, and get rid of the "little critic," which represents your inner thoughts or self-talk and tends to focus on the negatives and minimize the positives. The little critic uses negativity, which when left unresolved erodes trust and interpersonal relationships. Constructive feedback is an important part of team building, but it must be done tactfully within the social context of empathy and assertiveness, using responses such as: "How did you come to that conclusion?" "I'm a little confused; help me understand what you mean." and "Good point; I have some additional thoughts about that."

The team must also provide the following qualities for its members:

- *Feel potent or empowered*—Believe they can be effective and successful
- *Believe activities are meaningful and sanctioned by the organization*—Share common values and beliefs
- *Perform autonomously*—Freedom and discretion in directing goals/efforts
- *Perceive team results are valued and supported by the organization*—Recognize that their work impacts the organization (Fried, Topping, & Rundall, 2000)

Moreover, team tasks or goals must emphasize excellence and convey clear goals and expectations, match roles and training to level of complexity, define collaborative responsibilities, cross-train and learn each others' roles and responsibilities, establish a quality improvement process to evaluate team performance, and require cohesiveness when work is highly interdependent (Fried, et al., 2000). Collectively, these goals and membership qualities create a supportive environment of respect and collegiality for the frontline nurse leader and team members. They also help the nurse work more effectively within various social contexts, including clinical rounds, unit-based projects, and interdisciplinary teams (see Table 5-4).

Table 5-4 Ingredients for Team Success

- Recognition and reward for success
- Respect that involves praising publicly and criticizing privately
- Advice without reproach
- Acceptance and encouragement of members' creativity
- Active listening skills
- Empathy
- Assertiveness and conflict resolution skills
- Open dialogue among team members
- A focus on common concerns and issues
- Support of common interests
- Willingness to listen to the other side and encourage questions
- Present your position frankly and honestly, and respect the rights of others
- Silence (more eloquent than speech)
- Trusting and supportive work relationships
- Environment that encourages participation in the decision-making process
- Motivation, rejuvenation, inspiration, and fun

Despite understanding the importance of team-building skills and quality interpersonal relationships, nurses, who are predominantly women, continue to struggle with relational and gender issues. Studies indicate that women attach a greater emphasis to relationships than men and often link their self-esteem and self-worth to social contacts (Ballou, Bowers, Boyatzis, & Kolb, 1999; Carroll, 2005; Kram & Hall, 1996). Power exists in quality relationships with others, especially when there is strong mutual trust and a willingness to rely on each other for honest and constructive feedback. Cultivating healthy relationships affords a safe and high-quality social context in which nurses can both nurture and mentor their young and experienced colleagues and affirm their contributions to health care—key issues for healthy team building. More importantly, nurse–nurse relationships instill the confidence, trustworthiness, personal integrity, and optimism to embrace change; facilitate personal and professional development; and work effectively with others. Unfortunately, this level of trust and social context continues to elude many nurses and jeopardize their potential shared power base. Ideally, nurses must galvanize their own strengths and potentials and work collectively to establish team-building skills among themselves as a conduit to establish quality relationships with interdisciplinary team members.

Effective interdisciplinary teams afford opportunities for members to safely express personal opinions, share expertise, and respect others' input with the sole purpose of providing individualized care over the health care continuum. Nurses must be willing to ask the right questions, strengthen nurse–client relationships, and be mindful of obligations to employ holistic interventions and value difference in clients and colleagues. Because of individual differences and perspectives, conflict must be expected and dealt with effectively during interdisciplinary team meetings. Active listening and empathy or appreciation of others' perspectives facilitate healthy work relationships and advance the needs of staff while allowing a greater focus on client-centered health care and positive clinical outcomes. The following strategies also facilitate effective dialogue between the nurse and teams members faced with numerous challenges, such as reduced resources and staffing and higher client acuity:

- Listen to understand and glean the views and interests of others.
- Use open-ended questions.
- Employ reflective listening.
- Summarize.
- Cope with resistance.
- Value and be mindful of the rights of yourself and others.
- Build winning alliances.
- Assess the best approach and alternatives.
- Use creative cooperation.
- Employ effective negotiation skills.
- Be comfortable in an environment of change and transition.
- Remain calm during heated discussions.
- Be open to new ideas.
- Avoid personalizing disagreements.
- Think outside of the box.
- Look at the "big picture."

Acquisition of team-building skills enables the student, novice, and experienced nurse to enter collaborative relationships as active participants and decision makers. Besides effective communication skills, the nurse must become an expert in conflict management and negotiation. Collectively, team-building skills help nurses broker and advocate for safe and quality health care.

Interdisciplinary Teams

Advances in health and information technologies require sound clinical judgment and psychosocial skills. Integrating research and information technologies requires approaches that maximize resources, leadership skills, and collaborative relationships. Interdisciplinary team approaches to the delivery of health care have always been important. Interdisciplinary or interprofessional groups now are being used more extensively in health care as a means of solving health care problems, coordinating care across the continuum, managing complex client problems and needs, and optimizing health care (Fried, et al., 2000).

The ANA (2003) advocates nurses' involvement in shared decision making to ensure appropriate and timely response to human needs and societal expectations. The ANA defines three levels of work relationships. The first involves one person commanding another, the second is described as détente, and the third is collaboration. Nurses must assess and understand the different levels of work relationships with clients, families, colleagues, communities, and society. The first level is outdated and suggests that decisions are made by one person and exclusively followed by another. Realistically, in all work relationships individuals have to use their own knowledge and make sound clinical judgments. The second level, détente, requires involved parties to have an understanding and acknowledge mutual and shared goals and interests but this may mean that one person has more power than the other (both agree to disagree with respect for each other). Finally, the third level, collaboration, represents a true partnership where both parties share equal, shared power. Ideally, this level promotes a climate of mutual trust and respect and recognition of individual strengths and uniqueness. Although the third level is ideal, it rarely transpires. Growing tension continues to mount between nurses and other clinicians within the social context of changing health care systems, rising client acuity, and dwindling resources. Effective resolution of these issues is determined by the quality of communication and leadership skills necessary to resolve complex care issues while maintaining sound interpersonal relationships.

Successful teams value collaboration, respect each member's uniqueness and clinical expertise, and establish team processes that facilitate clear and open communication (Donaldson & Mohr, 2000). Members address clinical issues, resource allocation, and establish performance or quality improvement measures and maintain a forum in which to educate and coach others. The core of successful teams is effective communication among disciplines. Nurses play key roles on interdisciplinary teams and must be prepared to communicate effectively through education about teams and goal attainment (Antai-Otong, 1997).

Selective team membership is important to successful goal attainment. The selection of each team member must be based on the following:

- Right member
- Right size
- Right task/assignment
- Right attitude
- Right expertise

Goals galvanize teams and move them beyond individual agendas to client and organization goals. Factors that influence the effectiveness of interdisciplinary teams involve:

- Trust and genuine respect for members
- Open communication
- Collaboration
- Genuine interest in members
- Commitment to goals
- Membership involvement
- Respect and value of each member regardless of educational preparation or status
- Sense of ownership
- Respect for leaders
- Conflict resolution
- Learning from failures
- Team-defined rewards
- Problem solving and goal achievement
- Support from organizational hierarchies
- Collective (versus individual) responsibilities for goal achievement

Finally, the efficiency of interdisciplinary teams depends on trust, the quality of interpersonal relationships, being mindful of the uniqueness of each member, high-quality communication skills, and ultimately group cohesiveness (Antai-Otong, 1997). Regardless of specialty, education, and clinical background, nurses are pivotal members of interdisciplinary teams. Effective team participation requires assertive communication skills, motivation, a willingness to work and collaborate with others, and active involvement in the decision-making processes.

Quality health care evolves from nursing care provided 24 hours a day, 7 days a week during hospitalization. Consequently, bedside and frontline nurses must be prepared to participate in decision-making processes governing health care within interdisciplinary teams. Data gathered through the assessment and evaluation process, treatment implementation, and monitoring of client responses are invaluable to interdisciplinary treatment planning. The nurse's input must be clearly communicated based on critical thinking skills that guide interpersonal relationships with clients, families, and colleagues as well as health care planning and outcomes.

Individual barriers to effective team participation include lack of knowledge, low self-esteem, lack of confidence, poor interpersonal and communication skills, and ineffective conflict resolution skills. Barriers associated with teams as a whole include:

- Lack of respect for members
- Members focusing on individual needs instead of the team
- Unclear goals and objectives
- Lack of organization support (e.g., visibility, resources, time)
- Personality conflicts
- Poor leadership
- Lack of team trust
- Resistance to change
- Lack of respect or empathy
- Territorial issues between disciplines
- Intimidation
- Conflict of interest

Understanding the dynamics of team evolution and normal behaviors within the team promotes a greater understanding of each member's role in creating an effective team. Tuckerman (1965) delineated four stages of team development (see Table 5-5):

- *Forming*—Initial interactions with team members or the "honeymoon period."
- *Storming*—Turbulence and increased tension among members; goals are blurred; hidden agendas emerge.
- *Forming*—Members coalesce under effective leadership; members feel less threatened.
- *Performing*—Members perform at their peak; quality decision making and personal growth occur.

Knowledge of how teams form and perform combined with the recipe for team success enhances understanding of how the nurse can effectively

Table 5-5 Developmental Stages of Teams

Stage	Characteristics
Forming	Team members seek acceptance from others. The ability to work through this stage is governed by personal confidence, self-esteem, interpersonal and communication skills, a willingness to participate, emotional maturity, and creativity. This period is often referred to as the "honeymoon period," and is marked by excessive friendlessness and nonthreatening interactions. Questions are raised about team goals, resources, time frames, roles, strengths, and limitations.
Storming	This stage is filled with turbulence and stress as members become more task-oriented. Team resilience is tested as tensions mount, trust becomes uncertain, and hidden agendas emerge along with personality conflicts. Conflict resolution and assertiveness are imperative to maintain team stability. Resolution depends upon the quality of leadership—clear directions facilitate this process.
Norming	This stage is heralded by resolution of conflicts and disputes generated in the storming stage. Members begin to accept roles and responsibilities, relationships coalesce, and member strengths and limitations are accepted. Members become goal-directed and productive, and confident in the process.
Performing	This is the final stage of team development. Productivity increases. Internal conflicts are resolved. Earnest commitment and pride emerge. Team performance peaks. Resources are allocated appropriately. Quality decision making occurs.

work with others to establish goals and responsibilities and move toward quality shared decision making and implementation of evidence-based care.

In summary, nurses and other members of the interdisciplinary team must ensure cooperation between health professionals, integrate seamless expertise, and facilitate the appropriate exchange of information and care coordination across the health care continuum (IOM, 2001). Nurses can maximize team efforts by actively participating in team processes, sharing their expertise and clinical opinions, and strategizing to promote client-centered health care. Ideally, the nurse should have team-building skills, but these skills can be acquired through on-the-job training or mentoring.

PUBLIC SPEAKING SKILLS

As this chapter comes to a close, it is important to include the topic of public speaking or doing presentations as an essential leadership and communication skill. For a nurse to become an effective leader, he or she must be prepared to communicate effectively as a presenter or public speaker. Doing presentations in front of peers, colleagues, and professional meetings often generates tremendous anxiety and distress. Anxiety related to public speaking is common. A large number of people experience enormous distress due to performance or social anxiety. Even the most experienced public speakers and entertainers feel stage fright, and yes, they have to work at it, too. Fears of embarrassment or humiliation or just falling flat on one's face can be quite frightening. Nonetheless, the good news is that unless these reactions are debilitating there is little cause for alarm. Through public speaking and practice you can obviate anxiety and effectively manage your fears.

Stage fright or performance anxiety is associated with the way we think and perceive ourselves, others, and the world. Common misperceptions that stifle presenters include:

- You have to have an innate talent to be a good speaker.
- Other people can do it so easily.
- Good speakers can speak with little preparation.
- Experienced speakers are always calm.
- People would realize how nervous I am.
- Who wants to hear what I have to say?

Remember, these are common *misperceptions*. The reality is that public speaking is a learned skill that takes time, practice, and creativity. Most experts will tell you they, too, experience anxiety at times, but have overcome it and become great national and international public speakers. Comparing yourself to others is unfair because everyone has to begin somewhere and all are challenged to explore and develop the best approach for themselves. What works for one speaker may be a disaster for someone else. It is important to develop your own comfort zone. Public speaking improves with time, confidence, and expertise. You must plan, organize, deliver, interact, and follow up. The following steps are useful in developing public speaking skills:

- Start small—take on a small project, such as presenting a case study during a treatment planning meeting.
- Select a topic of interest and in your area of expertise.

- Know your material and be prepared, using established skills. Do the literature search and make sure your facts are accurate.
- Use legible professional audiovisuals (e.g., PowerPoint, handouts).
- Know the purpose of your speech.
- Practice the presentation or do a "dry run."
- Depending on the amount of material you plan to present, start small (e.g., 15- to 30-minute presentation).
- Use note cards or whatever audiovisual aids you prefer.
- Communicate the importance of your presentation.
- Prepare for questions.
- Enjoy your presentation.

Anxiety is common, so learn how to manage it—take slow, deep abdominal breaths and control your breathing. Pay attention to your respirations and use them as a way to reduce your heart rate, get centered, and "ground" yourself. This will come in handy when you actually present. The following section provides instruction on performing a deep breathing exercise.

Deep Breathing Exercise: Gain Control over Stage Fright

Once you decide on your format and how long to speak, it's time to practice. Begin by standing in front of a mirror and paying attention to nonverbal cues, such as excessive blinking, sweating, increased respirations, and lightheadedness. Get control of your physiological responses by taking 10 deep breaths using your abdominal muscles. Close your eyes and breathe slowly. Pay attention to your diaphragm by inhaling and pulling in your abdomen as your chest rises. Slowly release the breath and inhale again. Note how your respirations decrease along with your heart rate. (This is a very useful exercise that can be used with your eyes open or closed.) Once you feel relaxed, open you eyes and look in the mirror again and note the change in your nonverbal or body language. Do you feel calmer, more relaxed? If not, repeat this exercise. Now use your index cards to guide your practice run. Begin to speak; pay attention to physiological changes and use the deep breathing exercises to control both respirations and heart rate as needed. Controlling your physiological responses improves concentration and thought processes. Complete your practice run.

During the actual presentation, pay attention to your body and gain control as previously mentioned using deep abdominal breathing exercises. Focus on the message, not what others think of you. Visualize your success and focus on two or three friendly faces during your presentation. Once you complete the presentation, seek genuine feedback. Avoid personalizing constructive feedback and use it to improve your next presentation. Professional development and leadership skills require lifelong learning, and each presentation provides an opportunity to sharpen your creativity, clinical knowledge base, and communication skills. A prerequisite to personal growth and development is taking risks. You *must* be willing to step outside the box, take risks, and grow from each experience. The most successful leaders are also good communicators and public speakers.

Major advantages of public speaking skills include:

- Increase self-confidence
- Aid in pursuit of professional and career development
- Facilitate reporting the status of projects to colleagues, peers, and management
- Strengthen interpersonal communication with peers, clients, families, and management
- Increase visibility in your organization, particularly among professional colleagues

Public speaking is an important leadership and communication skill. Predictably, nurses who fail to develop this skill find themselves disappointed in career and professional advancement within their organizations. A solution to this challenge is finding several mentors who offer learning opportunities to sharpen your competence and confidence as a public speaker. Each event will motivate you to do more and enhance your self-esteem as a communicator and effective leader.

SELF-RENEWAL: THE FORGOTTEN LEADERSHIP COMPETENCE

The previous discussions focused on important leadership and communication skills, but it would be imprudent to omit a dialogue about self-renewal as part of effective leadership and professional development. The daily hassles of today's nurses are profound and are often overlooked. Historically, nurses have found it easier to take care of others, at the expense of taking care of themselves. Modern-day nurse leaders must create healing environments that extend beyond clients, families, and colleagues and include themselves to maintain emotional, physical, social, and spiritual health and overall well-being. As students, novices, and experienced nurses face the challenge of dwindling resources, inadequate staffing, and increased client acuity, they must make their personal health and self-renewal a priority. While focusing on leadership and communication development, nurses must also integrate and emulate the health behaviors they instill in their clients.

Recognizing personal and work-related stressors begins the self-renewal process. What are the most stressful things in your personal life?

- Caring for aging parents?
- Dealing with "normal" adolescent behavior?
- Experiencing marital discord?
- Dealing with mounting debts?
- Suffering from a chronic, acute, or debilitating emotional or medical problem?

How are you handling personal stressors? Do you communicate with others to sort out your feelings? Or do you keep things inside? Do you have stress-related health problems, such as hypertension, tension headaches, obesity or GI disturbances, or depression? Stress may not be the primary cause of such illnesses, but left unmanaged they can be debilitating or even life threatening. Answering these questions helps assess the nature of personal stressors that surely impact the way you feel about yourself, others, and the world; communicate with others; and care for yourself and clients.

The next step is to determine what types of work-related stressors you have. Are you:

- Experiencing interpersonal conflicts?
- Dealing with burnout?
- Loathing your job and where you are in your career?
- Making unnecessary errors or mistakes?
- Wishing you could retire today?
- Having difficulty finding positive things or pleasure in your job?

Again, similar to coping and dealing with personal stressors, unmanaged workplace stress eventually results in major medical and emotional problems simply because they go unrecognized or minimized. Self-renewal is the answer to these problems and requires high self-worth and self-esteem and a willingness to change.

Self-renewal must be a daily ritual that begins with a positive attitude about yourself, others, and the world. Positive self-talk such as "I am so glad I am alive and my day is going to be positive" and "I control how I react to personal and workplace stress" along with a positive attitude set the tone for the entire day. Assertiveness, conflict management, and even negotiation play key roles in how the nurse handles personal and job-related situations.

No one has control of external events, but believing that you have control of thoughts, feelings, and behaviors fosters a sense of control and empowerment. The opposite engenders feelings of powerlessness, anger, depression, and apathy. Self-renewal is the glue that maintains stability, integrity, health, and self-actualization. Each nurse must identify areas of interest and establish a daily self-renewal and health promotion agenda that incorporates the following five aspects of health:

- *Physical*—Getting an annual physical examination; healthy eating habits; regular exercise; planning and taking vacations at least once a year; regular dental appointments; age-related health examinations; monthly self-breast examinations; taking prescription medications as ordered; following treatment recommendations; using "mental health days" to recharge; taking bubble baths; relaxing in a Jacuzzi; getting regular manicures, pedicures, facials, and massages; taking regular lunch breaks; and getting adequate sleep
- *Mental*—Journaling, reading a good book, writing poetry, having several hobbies, allowing time for fun and relaxation
- *Psychological*—Thinking positive thoughts; focusing on the glass being half full rather than half empty; maintaining control over your feelings, thoughts, and behaviors through assertiveness; saying "no" without feeling overwhelmingly guilty; recognizing your strengths and limitations
- *Social*—Surrounding yourself with positive people; going to movies or art shows; biking; skiing; leaning on others in time of need
- *Spiritual*—Regular walks in the park, participating in religious rituals or prayers, sorting out "your purpose in life," letting go of anger

Effective leaders require the mental and physical stamina to lead. Without self-renewal, leadership and communication skills will be compromised or eroded. Professional development requires an action plan or daily agenda that integrates effective communication skills to enhance quality interpersonal and work relationships with lifelong learning. This chapter has integrated these principles, and challenges students and nurses to make the best of their personal lives and careers through daily self-renewal activities.

SUMMARY

This chapter has described the major elements of effective leadership and professional development. It is clear that self-awareness, self-renewal, lifelong learning, cultural sensitivity, and a plurality of communication skills are essential for effective leadership. Leadership exists in every hierarchy within the organization, from the novice to the experienced nurse; on the frontline and in the boardroom. Regardless of leadership role, communication is a core requirement that enables the nurse to share relevant clinical information to the interdisciplinary team, provide quality health education to clients and families, and present current research during a case study.

Leadership and communication skills determine the nurse's level of effectiveness and lifelong learning and professional development. The real value of leadership as a novice or experienced nurse is not where you begin, but where you finish. Regardless of position in the organization, nurses are leaders and must be prepared to embrace their responsibilities as brokers of client-centered care across the health care continuum. Failure to accept these responsibilities, as evidenced by ineffective communication and poor leadership skills, keeps the nurse out of healing relationships. Critical communication skills empower the nurse to lead, to advocate for safe and quality care, and to actively participate in shared decision making with clients, families, and interdisciplinary teams.

Today's nurse must be emotionally and physically fit to cope with the daily hassles of providing care for complex health problems and meeting the individual needs of their clients. Although self-renewal is sometimes minimized and overlooked it must be an integral part of the nurse's daily rituals.

SUGGESTIONS FOR CLINICAL AND EXPERIENTIAL ACTIVITIES

1. Ask one of the frontline nurse leaders to allow you to shadow him or her during two interdisciplinary meetings and discuss the team's developmental stage. Present your findings to the class.
2. Do a 5-minute "soap box" presentation on a relevant clinical topic. Seek feedback on your public speaking.
3. Interview a nurse executive to discuss how he or she was promoted and characteristics of effective leadership and developmental skills, including conflict resolution and negotiation.
4. Interview a frontline nurse to discuss his or her personal and professional development plans and how they fit into the goals and mission of the organization.
5. Interview a psychiatric advanced practice nurse or other professional to learn how to do deep breathing exercises in preparation for presentations and other stressful situations. Create a presentation on this technique and present it to the class.

END-OF-CHAPTER QUESTIONS

1. Emotional intelligence is an important leadership quality. All of the following are characteristics of emotional intelligence *except:*
   a. Enhances self-awareness of emotional responses to given situations.
   b. Increases intelligence that facilitates problem solving.
   c. Improves interpersonal relationships by reducing emotions.
   d. Increases sensitivity and awareness of others' needs.

2. Client-centered health care refers to:
   a. Integrating the client's decisions, needs, and wishes into care.
   b. Collaborating with the client and family.
   c. Making the client the center of treatment planning.
   d. All of the above.

3. Which of the following statements best describes assertiveness?
   a. I was offended by the way you yelled in front of the client.
   b. You make me angry every time you yell at me in front of others.
   c. I am sorry I upset you and made you yell.
   d. You are so difficult to work with because of your attitude.

4. Which of the following is the most accurate statement about conflicts?
   a. They are a natural part of relationships.
   b. They must be avoided at all costs.
   c. They stem from poor communication skills.
   d. It's easier to walk away and let the conflicts resolve themselves.

5. Forming is one of the stages of team development. Which of the following best describes this stage?
   a. Team members are able to make quality decisions.
   b. Team members are trying to understand others and their roles.
   c. Teams members experience turbulence and high tension.
   d. Team members distrust each other and hidden agendas emerge.

6. Team members have met several times. During the current meeting, the physician points out that nurse Jackson is disrupting the meeting because she asks too many questions and is unwilling to follow instructions. What does the physician's behavior reflect?
   a. A failure to appreciate and respect the nurse's expertise and opinion.
   b. A strong leadership role.
   c. Assertive communication techniques.
   d. A clear delineation of the physician's and nurse's role on the team.

7. Trust plays a pivotal role in team building. Which of the following demonstrates team trust?
   a. I disagree with you and feel this is a better solution.
   b. I prefer to keep my ideas to myself.

    c. Your ideas are always inappropriate.

    d. Let's talk about something else. This is too stressful.

8. Public speaking is a necessary leadership and communication skill. When preparing for a presentation, what is the most important consideration?

    a. Present on topics related to your expertise and interests.

    b. Select a topic your supervisor suggests despite your lack of expertise.

    c. Practice is unnecessary because it won't lower your anxiety.

    d. Limit your presentations to the unit level until your anxiety abates.

9. The *primary* benefit of interdisciplinary teams is improved work relationships.

    a. True

    b. False

Answers

1. b
2. d
3. a
4. a
5. b
6. a
7. a
8. a
9. False

Research Study 5–1

Title: Organizational Attributes Valued by Hospital, Home Care, and District Nurses in the United States and New Zealand. Flynn, L., Carryer, J., & Budge, C. (2005). *Journal of Nursing Scholarship, 37,* 67–72.

Purpose: This study was conducted to compare responses from hospital-based, home care, and district registered nurses in the United States to responses from nurses in New Zealand concerning the degree to which organizational attributes shown in the Nursing Work Index-Revised (NWI-R) were valued as important to the support of their professional practice.

Method: Researchers surveyed 403 home care nurses in the United States and 320 nurses in New Zealand from a pool with an existing data set of 669 hospital-based nurses to conduct this descriptive and nonexperimental study. The NWI-R was used to measure the presence of organizational attributes that comprised a professional nursing practice environment. Data were analyzed by frequency distributions and analysis of variance.

Results/Findings: Approximately 80% of hospital-based, home care, and district nurses exhibited a high degree of agreement that 47 out of 49 items on the NWI-R were organizational attributes relevant to the support of their professional practice. Researchers recommended further research to identify key organizational characteristics that allow predicting positive nurse and client outcomes in these settings.

Implications for Nurses: Organizational attributes play significant roles in professional nurse development. The NWI-R lists qualities described in this chapter that advance the role of nurses and professional development—autonomy, control of practice, physician relationships, and organizational support. As previously discussed, effective communication and quality interpersonal relationships are critical skills for today's nurse and promote a sense of autonomy, control of practice, job satisfaction, and confidence in a changing health care system.

Research Study 5–2

Title: Linking the Practice Environment to Nurses' Job Satisfaction Through Nurse-Physician Communication. Manojlovich, M. (2005). *Journal of Nursing Scholarship, 37,* 367–373.

Purpose: The investigator explored the direct and indirect association between practice environment, nurse-physician (RN-MD) communication, job-satisfaction, as it hypothesized in the nursing role effectiveness model (NREM).

Method/Design: The investigator used a nonexperimental survey design. Her sample (n=500) consisted of acute care nurses obtained from a list from the Michigan Nurses Association. Nurses in the sample had to be currently employed, work in hospital, and working as either a staff nurse or had regular direct patient contact. Study instruments were the Conditions for Work Effectiveness Questionnaire-II (CWEQ-II), the Practice Environment Scale of the Nursing Work Index (PES-NWI), the ICU Nurse-Physician Questionnaire, and the Index of Work Satisfaction (IWS), Part B. Inferential statistical tests included multiple regression, *t*-tests and one-way analysis of variance (ANOVA). Out of the 500 packets used to survey nurses, 332 were returned with 316 used in the study.

Results/Findings: Major findings from this study indicated that the practice environment and structural empowerment scales predicted both nursing job satisfaction and the quality of RN-MD communication.

Implications for Nurses

As mentioned earlier in this chapter, nurse leaders must create and adopt proactive strategies to shore up social support and job satisfaction by developing and implementing initiatives that empower nurses to develop and utilize effective communication. Equally important is the need for nurses to nurture their newest colleagues and to support experienced nurses to enhance RN-MD work relationships and retain quality nursing staff.

REFERENCES

AbuAlRub, R. F. (2004). Job stress, job performance, and social support among hospital nurses. *Journal of Nursing Scholarship, 36,* 73–78.

Aiken, L. H., Clarke, S. P., Sloan, D. M., Sochalski, J., & Silber, J. H. (2002). Hospital nurse staffing and patient mortality, burnout and job satisfaction. *Journal of the American Medical Association, 288,* 1987–1993.

American Nurses Association. (2003). *Nursing's social policy statement* (2nd ed.). Washington, DC: Author.

American Nurses Association. (2004). *Nursing: Scope and standards of practice.* Washington, DC: Author.

American Nurses Credentialing Center. (2005). Magnet recognition program. Retrieved September 10, 2005, from http://www.nursingworld.org/ancc/magnet/benes.html

Antai-Otong, D. (1997). Team building in a health care setting. *American Journal of Nursing, 97,* 48–51.

Antai-Otong, D. (1999). Continued professional development. In C. A. Shea, L. R. Peller, E. C. Poster, G. W. Stuart, & M. P. Verhey (Eds.), *Advanced Practice Nursing in Psychiatric and Mental Health Care* (pp. 467–480). St. Louis: Mosby Publising.

Antai-Otong, D. (2001). Creative stress-management for self-renewal. *Dermatology Nursing, 13,* 31–32, 35–39.

Antai-Otong, D. (2002). Culturally sensitive treatment of African Americans with substance-related disorders. *Journal of Psychosocial Nursing, 40,* 1–6.

Arora, N. K., & McHorney, C. A. (2000). Patient preferences for medical decision making: Who really wants to participate? *Medical Care, 36,* 325–341.

Ballou, R., Bowers, D., Boyatzis, R. E., & Kolb, D. A. (1999). Fellowship in lifelong learning: An executive development program for professionals. *Journal of Management Education, 23,* 338–354.

Beach, M. C., Sugarman, J., Johnson, R. L., Arbelaez, J. J., Duggan, P. S., & Cooper, L. A. (2005). Do patients treated with dignity report higher satisfaction, adherence, and receipt of preventive care? *Annals of Family Medicine, 3,* 331–338.

Bennis, W., & Townsend, R. (1995). *Reinventing leadership.* New York: Quill/ William Morrow.

Betancourt, J. R. (2004). Cultural competence—marginal or mainstream movement. *New England Journal of Medicine, 351,* 953–955.

Bower, S. A., & Bower, G. H. (1976). *Asserting self.* Reading, MA: Addison-Wesley.

Bulger, R. J. (2000). The quest for the therapeutic organization. *Journal of the American Medical Association, 283,* 2431–2433.

Campinha-Bacote, J. (1999). *The process of cultural competence in the delivery of health care services: A culturally competent model of care* (3rd ed.). Cincinnati, OH: Transcultural C.A.R.E Associates.

Carrillo, J. E., Green, A. G., & Betancourt, J. R. (1999). Cross-cultural primary care: A patient-based approach. *Annals of Internal Medicine, 130,* 829–834.

Carroll, T. L. (2005). Leadership skills and attributes of women and nurse executives: Challenges for the 21st century. *Nursing Administration Quarterly, 29,* 146–153.

Clark, N. M., Janz, N. K., Dodge, J. A., Schork, M. A., Fingerlin, T. E., Wheeler, J. R., et al. (2000). Changes in functional status of older women with heart disease: Evaluation of a program based on self-regulation. *Journals of Gerontology Series B Psychological Social Science, 55,* S117–S123.

Crawley, L., Marshall, P., & Koenig, B. (2001). *Respecting cultural differences at the end of life.* Philadelphia: American College of Physicians, American Society of Internal Medicine.

Daiski, I. (2004). Changing nurses' disempowering relationship patterns. *Journal of Advanced Nursing, 48,* 43–50.

Donaldson, M. S., & Mohr, J. J. (2000). *Exploring innovation and quality improvement in health care micro-systems: A cross-case analysis.* Washington, DC: Institute of Medicine, National Academy Press.

Edwards, A., Elwyn, G., Hood, K., Atwell, C., Robling, M., Houston, H., et al. (2004). Patient-based outcome results from a cluster randomized trial of shared decision making skills development and use of risk communication aids in general practice. *Family Practice, 21,* 347–354.

Freeman, L. H., & Adams, P. F. (1999). Comparative effectiveness of two nursing programmes on assertive behaviour. *Nursing Standard, 38,* 23–35.

Freshman, B., & Rubino, L. (2002). Emotional intelligence: A core competency for health care administrators. *Health Care Management, 20,* 1–9.

Fried, B. J., Topping, S., & Rundall, T. G. (2000). Groups and teams in health services organizations. In S. M. Shortell & A. D. Kaluzny (Eds.), *Health Care Management: Organization Design and Behavior* (4th ed., Chapter 6). Albany, NY: Delmar.

Goleman, D. (1996). *Emotional intelligence.* London, England: Bloomsbury.

Goleman, D. (1998). *Working with emotional intelligence.* New York: Bantam.

Goleman, D., Boyatzis, R., & McKee, A. (2003). *Primal leadership: Realizing the power of emotional intelligence.* Boston: Harvard Business School Press.

Harrison, A. (2000). Choice is a gift from the patient to the doctor, not the other way around [Letter]. *British Medical Journal, 320,* 874.

Healy, C., & McKay, M. (2000). Nursing stress: The effects of coping strategies and job satisfaction in a sample of Australian nurses. *Journal of Advanced Nursing, 31,* 681–688.

Herbert, R., & Edgar, L. (2004). Emotional intelligence: A primal dimension of nursing leadership. *Canadian Journal of Nursing Leadership, 17,* 56–63.

Humphreys, J., Brunsen, B., & Davis, D. (2005). Emotional structure and commitment: Implications for health care management. *Journal of Health and Organizational Management, 19,* 120–129.

Institute of Medicine. (2001). *Crossing the quality chasm. A new health system for the 21st century.* Washington, DC: National Academy Press.

Kane, D., & Thomas, B. (2000). Nursing and the "F" word. *Nursing Forum, 35,* 17–24.

Kram, K. E., & Hall, D. T. (1996). Mentoring in a context of diversity and turbulence. In E. E. Kossek & S. A. Lobel (Eds.), *Managing Diversity: Human Resource Strategies for Transforming the Workplace* (pp. 108–136). Cambridge, MA: Blackwell Business.

Kuokkanen, L., Leino-Kilpi, H., & Katajisto, J. (2003). Nurse empowerment, job satisfaction, and organizational commitment. *Journal of Nursing Care Quality, 18,* 184–192.

Lorig, K. R., Ritter, P., Stewart, A. L., Sobel, D. S., Brown, B. W. Jr., Bandura, A., et al. (2001). Chronic disease self-management program: 2-year health status and health utilization outcomes. *Medical Care, 39,* 1217–1223.

MacPhee, M., & Scott, J. (2002). The role of social support networks for rural hospital nurses: Supporting and sustaining the rural nursing work force. *The Journal of Nursing Administration, 32,* 264–272.

Mansell, D., Poses, R. M., Kazis, L., & Duefield, C. A. (2000). Clinical factors that influence patients' desire for participation in decisions about illness. *Archives of Internal Medicine, 160,* 2991–2996.

McQueen, A. C. H. (2004). Emotional intelligence in nursing work. *Journal of Advanced Nursing, 47,* 101–108.

Mills, J., Francis, K., & Bonner, A. (2005). Mentoring, clinical supervisions and preceptoring: Clarifying conceptual definitions for Australian rural nurses. A review of the literature. *Rural and Remote Journal, 5,* 410. Retrieved January 19. 2006, from http://rrh.deakin.edu.au/articshowarticlenewles/.asp?ArticleID=410

National Institute of Standards and Technology. (2000). Health care criteria for performance and excellence. Baldridge National Quality Program 2000. CARE

Baldridge Web site. Retrieved January 19, 2006, from http://www.quality.nist.gov/HealthCare_Criteria.htm

Nolan, M., Lundh, U., & Brown, J. (1999). Changing aspects of nurses' work environment: A comparison of perceptions in two hospitals in Sweden and UK and implications for recruitment of staff. *National Research, 4,* 221–234.

Paasche-Orlow, M. (2004). The ethics of cultural competence. *Academic Medicine, 79,* 347–350.

Porter-O'Grady, T., & Malloch, K. (2003). *Quantum leadership: A textbook of leadership.* Sudbury, MA: Jones and Bartlett.

Purnell, L. (2002). The Purnell model for cultural competence. *Journal of Transcultural Nursing, 13,* 193–196.

Purnell, L. D., & Paulanka, B. J. (2003). *Transcultural healthcare: A culturally competent approach* (2nd ed.). Philadelphia: F. A. Davis.

Reeves, A. (2005). Emotional intelligence: Recognizing and regulating emotions. *American Association of Occupational Health Nursing Journal, 53,* 172–176.

Rochester, S., Kilstoff, K., & Scott, G. (2005). Learning from success: Improving undergraduate education through understanding the capabilities of successful nurse graduates. *Nurse Education Today, 25,* 181–188.

Scott, C. J. (1997). Enhancing patient outcomes through an understanding of intercultural medicine: Guidelines for the practitioner. *Maryland Medical Journal, 46,* 175–180.

Skopec, W. M., & Kiely, L. S. (1994). *Everything is negotiable when you know how to play the game.* New York: American Management Association.

Smith, L. S. (1998). Concept analysis: Cultural competence. *Journal of Cultural Diversity, 5,* 4–10.

Stewart, M., Brown, J. B., Boon, H., Galajda, J., Meredith, L., & Sangster, M. (1999). Evidence on patient-doctor communication. *Cancer Prevention Control, 3,* 25–30.

Stiggelbout, A. M., & Kiebert, G. M. (1997). A role for the sick role. Patient preferences regarding information and participation in clinical decision-making. *Canadian Medical Association Journal, 157,* 383–389.

Tuckerman, B. (1965). Developmental sequences in small groups. *Psychological Bulletin, 63,* 384–399.

Veatch, R. (2000). *Cross-cultural perspectives in medical ethics.* Sudbury, MA: Jones and Bartlett.

Wade, G. H. (2004). A model of the attitudinal component of professional nurse autonomy. *Journal of Nurse Education, 43,* 116–124.

Welch, M. (1998). Required curricula in diversity and cross-cultural medicine: The time is now. *Journal of American Medical Women's Association, 53*(Suppl.), 121–123.

SELECTED WEB SITES

Advisory Commission on Consumer Protection and Quality in the Health Care Industry. Quality First: Better Health Care for All Americans: http://www.hcqualitycommission.gov/final

American Nurses Credentialing Center: http://www.nursingworld.org/ancc/

Baldrige National Quality Program. Health Care Criteria for Performance Excellence—Provides a systems perspective for understanding performance management http://www.quality.nist.gov/HealthCare_Criteria.htm

EthnoMed—Ethnic medicine information from Harborview Medical Center: http://www.ethnomed.org

Georgetown Center for Child and Human Development, National Center for Cultural Competence—Curricula Enhancement Module Series: http://www.nccccurricula.info

Georgetown Center for Child and Human Development, National Center for Cultural Competence—Cultural Competence Health Practitioner Assessment: https://www4.georgetown.edu/uis/keybridge/keyform/form.cfm?formID=277

Office of Minority Health Information Center. Assuring Cultural Competence in Health Care—Recommendations for National Standards and an Outcomes-Focused Research Agenda: http://www.omhrc.gov/clas

The Park Ridge Center for Health, Faith, and Ethics—Offers a series of books (*Health and Medicine in the Faith Traditions*) that provide general information about various religions: http://www.parkridgecenter.org

Robert Wood Johnson Publications and Resources. Cultural Transformation in Health Care: A white paper that describes the complex nature of organization and culture and its role in health care organization: http://www.rwjf.org/files/publications/NursingCulturalTrans.PDF

Index

Italicized page locators refer to a figure; tables are denoted with a *t*

A

Acceptance, 91
Access Project, Web site for, 51
Active listening, 29, 57–59, 91, 217
    barriers to, 59, 60*t*
    defined, 54
    successful negotiation and, 75
    team-building and, 220
    verbalizing the implied and, 83
AD. *See* Alzheimer's disease
ADHD. *See* Attention deficit/hyperactivity
    disorder
Administration on Aging—How to Find Help,
    Web site for, 97
Administration on Aging Resources for
    Minorities and Diverse Populations, Web
    site for, 192
Adolescence
    communication during, 22–23
    nurse–client relationship and, 116
    therapeutic communication techniques
        and, 87–88
Adolescents
    confidentiality issues with, 37
    culture and communication and, 174–176
    dying or seriously ill, end-of-life
        communication and, 125–131
    seriously ill, coping reactions in, 128*t*
Advance directives
    palliative care and, 124
    planning for, 123–124
    transcultural care and, 183

Advisory Commission on Consumer Protection
    and Quality in the Health Care Industry,
    Web site for, 238
Affect, 17
Age, health care disparities and, 165
Ageism, 89, 118, 165
Agency for Healthcare Research and Quality,
    Web site for, 152
Aggressive behaviors, nurse–client relationship
    and, 32–33
Aggressive communication, assertive
    communication *vs.,* 60–61, 61*t*
Aggressive situations, nurse responding to
    (example), 65
Alzheimer's Association, Web site for,
    151
Alzheimer's Association Diversity Toolbox,
    Web site for, 151
Alzheimer's disease, 14
    communication and, 25, 26
American Academy of Pediatrics, Web site for,
    151
American Nurses Association, 205, 221
    Code of Ethics for Nurses, 36
American Nurses Credentialing Center, 205
    Web site for, 238
American Translators Association, Web site
    for, 192
ANA. *See* American Nurses Association
ANCC. *See* American Nurses Credentialing
    Center
Anger
    acknowledging, 31

assertiveness and, 63
emotional competence and, 17
Anxiety
impact of, on nurse–client relationship, 31–33
public speaking and, 226–227
Aphasias, 2, 12–13
Assertive communication
comparison of aggressive communication, passive communication and, 61*t*
health education and, 178–179
specific patterns of, 208*t*
Assertiveness, 59–61, 63–66, 91, 197
defined, 54, 196
professional, 206–207
essential characteristics of, 207*t*
setting stage for, 63–66
Association of Telehealth Service Providers, The, Web site for, 97
Attachment, 2, 16
Attachment theory, 2, 16, 20
Attention deficit/hyperactivity disorder, 14
Auditory cortex, role of, 12
Auditory hallucinations, in schizophrenia, 14, 15
Autism, 12, 15
Autism Spectrum Disorders (Pervasive Developmental Disorders), Web site for, 51
Autonomy, defined, 196

B

Baldrige National Quality Program, Web site for, 238
Beliefs, 154, 155
Bennis, W., 201
Berlo, D. K., 7
Bias, 19, 118
evidence of, 210
health care disparities and, 160
self-awareness and recognition of, 112, 165
Bipolar disorder, personal space issues and, 35
Body language, 2, 5, 33, 54
assertiveness and, 65
caring for dying or seriously ill child or adolescent and, 127
effective communication and, 202
Boundaries, professional, 39–41

Bowlby, J., 16
Boyatzis, R., 200
Brain, regions of, involved in speech, *11*, 11–12
Broca's area, of brain, 2, *11*, 12, 13
Burnout, 202

C

Cain, J. M., 177
Campinha-Bacote, J., 155
Care coordination home telehealth, 110, 111
Career development, 204
Caregiver strain, 139
CCHT. *See* Care coordination home telehealth
Cellular phones, 4, 22, 38
Cerebral hemispheric dominance, language and, 10
Chat rooms, 4, 22
CHID. *See* Combined Health Information Database
Child abuse
disclosure and, 37
duty to warn or inform and, 39
Childhood
communication during, 22
nurse–client relationships and, 114–115
therapeutic communication techniques and, 84–85
Children. *See also* Parents
confidentiality issues with, 37
culture and communication and, 174–176
dying or seriously ill, end-of-life communication and, 125–131
seriously ill, coping reactions in, 128*t*
Clarification, 66–67
defined, 54
example of, 66–67
Client-centered care, 101, 197
defined, 100
as innate right, 156
Closed-ended questioning, 77–79
example dialogue, 78
Cochrane Collaboration, Web site for, 152
Code of Ethics for Nurses (American Nurses Association), 36
Cognitive deficits, in Alzheimer's disease, 25

Collaboration. *See also* Teams
  defined, 100, 119–120
  ensuring quality in, 120
  systems thinking and, 205
Collaborative dialogue, example of, 120–121
Collaborative relationships, 119–122, 140
  with client and family, 119–121
  within interdisciplinary teams, 121–122
Combined Health Information Database, Web
  site for, 97
Communication. *See also* Communication
  theories; Cultural aspects of
  communication partnerships;
  Effective communication;
  Therapeutic communication.
  complexity of, 41
  culture's role in, 18–19
  defined, 2
  developmental/life span issues, 20–26
    adolescence, 22–23
    adulthood, 23
    infancy and childhood, 20–22
    older adulthood, 23–26
  effective
    attributes of, 202
    negotiation and, 216–217
  factors and trends associated with, 9–27
  fundamental importance of, 3
  modes of, 27–35
  neurobiology of, 10–11
  neurodevelopmental disorders and, 15
  nonverbal, 5, 54, 58
  psychosocial issues in, 15–18
  public speaking skills, 225–227
  sensory-perceptual influences on, 13–15
  societal and health care trends and, 26
  technological advances in, 4
  technological and information systems
    and, 26–27
Communication style, cultural competence
  and, 166–168
Communication theories, 5–9
  dyadic interpersonal communication
    model, 7
  experiential communication theories, 7–9
  Peplau's interpersonal relation theory, 6–7
Conference calls, 4

Confidentiality, 27, 36–37, 56, 109, 123
Conflict management, 68, 213–214
Conflict resolution, 67–69, 91
  defined, 54
  example dialogue, 68–69
Conflicts
  causes contributing to, 213
  defined, 54
  traits associated with, 67
Confrontation, 69–70
  defined, 54
  example dialogue, 70
Conger, K. J., 117
Congruency, 8
COPE. *See* Creating Opportunities for Parent
  Empowerment
Coping capabilities/reactions
  right hemisphere in brain and, 16
  in seriously ill children and adolescents,
    128*t*
Creating Opportunities for Parent
  Empowerment, 115
Creativity, negotiation and, 216
Credentialing, 205
Critically ill children, nurse–client relationship
  and, 114–115
Critical thinking questions
  appropriate response to older client's
    yelling, 90
  assertive, passive, and aggressive
    communication styles, 62
  communicating with ill Hispanic child
    and mother with limited English
    proficiency, 176–177
  conflict management, 214
  hospice setting life expectation questions,
    135
Crossing the Quality Chasm (Institute of
  Medicine), 197
Cultural aspects of communication
  partnerships, 153–184
  across the life span, 172–183
  changing demographics and, 157–159
  cultural competence and, 162–172
  health care disparities and, 159–162
  key terms related to, 154
  overview of, 154–157

Cultural competence, 155
  communication considerations and,
      162–172
  communication style and, 166–168
  defined, 154
  essential principles of, 211
  facilitating, 161
  self-awareness and, 165–166, 184
  shared decision making and, 210
  social organization and, 172
  space and, 170–172
  time and, 168–170
  uniqueness of parent–child interaction
      and, 176
Cultural sensitivity, 211
Cultural space
  appreciation of, 171
  defined, 154
Cultural values, within Sunrise Model, 163
Culture, 154
  dialogue illustrating impact of, on
      families, 181–182
  dying older adults and, 138
  older adulthood and, 89
  older adult's communication skills and,
      24, 25
  role of, in communication, 18–19
  shared decision making and, 209–212
  treatment planning and, 55
Culture and communication across life span,
    172–183
  assessment process, 173–174
  children and adolescents, 174–176
  families, 180–182
  gender sensitivity considerations
      (women), 177–180
  older adulthood, 182–183
Curanderos, 181
Customs, cultural context and, 167

D

Davidhizar, R. E., 172
Death and dying, communicating about, with
    children and adolescents, 129
Decision making, shared, 102, 122

Decoder, in dyadic interpersonal
    communication, 7, 7
Deep breathing exercises, 64t
  for gaining control over stage fright,
      226–227
Delusions, 14
Dementia, communication and, 25–26
Demographics, changing, 157–159
Depression, 14
  in stroke patients, 13
Despair, older adulthood and, 24, 89
Developmental issues, knowledge of, in caring
    for dying or seriously ill child or
    adolescent, 127
Dialogues
  client's threatening/aggressive behavior
      and nurse's response to, 32–33
  rapport fostered through, 28–29
Dignity, older adulthood and, 24
Disruptive behavior, workplace stress and, 4–5
Distance zones, 34
  across cultures, 170
Diversity
  communication and, 18–19
  nursing profession and, 158
  shared decision making and, 209–212
Documentation, legal and ethical
    considerations for, 38–39
Duty to protect third parties, 39
Dyadic interpersonal communication, 7, 7
DynaMed, Web site for, 152
Dyslexia, 13

E

Effective communication
  attributes of, 202
  factors related to, 27–28
  negotiation and, 216–217
Effective leaders, qualities in, 199–205
Effective leadership, core domains of, 200
Elder abuse, duty to warn or inform and, 39
Electronic medical records, 38, 110
Email, 4, 22, 56, 108
  benefits and liabilities with, 122–123
Emotional competence, 2, 17

Emotional intelligence, 200
  defined, 196
  Empathy, 2, 3
  defined, 100
  effective communication and, 30–31
  healing relationships and, 101
  team-building and, 220
Empowerment, defined, 196
EMR. *See* Electronic medical records
Encoder, in dyadic interpersonal
    communication, 7, 7
Encryption, 123
End-of-life care
  decision making and, 123
  holistic cultural needs and, 183
  self-awareness and, 112–113
End-of-life communication, 124–140
  with dying or seriously ill child or
      adolescent, 125–131
  in middle adulthood, 131–135
  in older adulthood, 135–140
  palliative care and, 124–125
  seven-step approach in, 132–133
Equitable health care, quality of care and, 162
Erikson, E. H., 29
Ethics, 56. *See also* Legal and ethical
    considerations
  dying older adults and, 138
  electronic messaging systems and, 109
Ethnicity, 156
  changing demographics and, 157
  defined, 154
  dying older adults and, 138
  health care disparities and, 159–162, 165
  nurse-client relationship and, 19
  older adulthood and, 89
  older adult's communication skills and,
      24, 25
  shared decision making and, 209–212
  treatment planning and, 55
Ethnohistory concepts, within Sunrise Model,
    163
EthnoMed, Web site for, 192, 238
Evidence-based care, technological support
    for, 198
Evidence-based decision making, defined, 196

Experiential communication theories, 7–9
Exploitation phase, in nurse–client
    relationship, 6, 107
Expressive (or nonfluent) aphasia, 12–13
Eye contact
  cultural competence and, 165, 166, 167
  effective communication and, 202
  good listening and, 58
  interactions with children and, 85
  trust and, 29

F

Facial markings, 167
Families. *See also* Children; Parents
  collaboration with, 119–121
  culture and communication and, 180–182
  death and dying of older adults and, 137
  dialogue illustrating impact of culture on,
      181–182
  dying or seriously ill child or adolescent
      and, 126–127
  nurse–client relationship and, 116–117
  shared decision making and, 208
  therapeutic communication and, 56,
      85–87
  therapeutic dialogue example, 86
Fax technology, 4
Fear, dying or seriously ill child or adolescent
    and, 128
Federal Interagency Forum on Age-Related
    Statistics, Older Americans, 2004, Web
    site for, 192
Firewalls, 123
Florida Initiative in Telehealth and Education
    (FITE), 108
Fluent aphasia, 12, 13
Focusing, 71–72
  defined, 54
  example dialogue, 71
Forming stage, in team development, 223, 224*t*
Frontal cortex, damage to or deficits in, 14

G

Gardner, J., 158

Gender
    health care disparities and, 160, 165
    sensitivity considerations for women,
        177–180
    team-building and, 219
Georgetown Center for Child and Human
    Development, National Center for
    Cultural Competence, Web sites for,
    192–193, 238
Giger, J. N., 172
Goleman, D., 200
Good listening, characteristics of, 58
Grief, dying or seriously ill child or adolescent
    and, 127
Grooming, within cultural context, 167

H

Hall, Edward T., 34, 170
Hallucinations, 14
Handheld computers, 38
Health care
    disparities in, 159–162
    information technology and advancement
        of, 56–57
    role of nurses and transitions in, 199
Health care disparities
    African Americans and, 183
    women and, 178
Health care systems, IOM recommendations
    on redesign of, 197–198
Health care trends, nurse–client relationships
    and, 26
Health education, 168
    assertive communication dialogue and,
        178–179
Health promotion, for nurses, 229
Healthy People 2010, 160
Hidden Dimension, The (Hall), 34, 170
HIPAA (Health Insurance Portability and
    Accountability Act of 1996), 109, 123
    Web site for, 151
Holistic assessment, of families and
    communities, 173–174
Holistic care, 101

Hope, dying or seriously ill child or adolescent
    and, 126
Hospice, 132
    defined, 100
Hospice Association of America, Web site for,
    151
Hospice Foundation of America, Web site for,
    152
Humor
    cultural context and, 168
    defined, 54
    effective leadership and, 204
    therapeutic qualities of, 73
Hygiene, within cultural context, 167

I

ICIC. *See* Improving Chronic Illness Care
Identification phase, in nurse–client
    relationship, 6, 106–107
Imparting information, 72–73
    defined, 54
    example dialogue, 72
Improving Chronic Illness Care, Web site for,
    152
Incongruent messages, 8
Infancy
    communication during, 20–21
    Latin root for, 84
    nurse–client relationships and, 114–115
    therapeutic communication techniques
        and, 84–85
Infant–primary caregiver relationship,
    attachment theory and, 15–16
Information technology
    security and, 38
    therapeutic communication and, 56
Insecure attachment styles
    in adulthood, 21
    interpersonal relationships and, 16–17
Institute of Medicine, 26, 110, 197
    Web site for, 152
Integrity
    effective leadership and, 204
    older adulthood and, 24, 89, 135

Interactive health communication, 122
Interdisciplinary collaboration, 4
    dying or seriously ill child or adolescent
        and, 126
Interdisciplinary teams, 121–122, 220–224,
    230
    cohesiveness and, 198
    factors influencing effectiveness of, 222
Internet, 27, 56, 168
    ethical concerns and, 109
    nurse–client relationships and, 108–109,
        111
    transcultural knowledge, peer
        collaboration and, 158, 159
Interpersonal relationships, secure attachment
    styles and, 16
Interpersonal Relations in Nursing (Peplau),
    6, 103, 114
Interpersonal skills, negotiation and, 74, 216
Intimate distance/close range distance zone,
    34, 170
IOM. *See* Institute of Medicine

J

Job satisfaction, 202
Jourard, S. M., 80

K

Kiely, L. S., 215
Kinship factors, within Sunrise Model, 163

L

Language, 2
    development of, during early childhood,
        21
    disorders of, 12–13
    neurobiology of, 10–11
    within Sunrise Model, 163
Language barriers, consequences of, 162–163
Language problems, early identification of, 22
Laughter, therapeutic qualities of, 73
Leaders, self-renewal and, 227–229

Leadership, effective, core domains of, 200
Leading, through effective communication,
    195–230
Learning disorders, 12–13, 13
Left hemisphere of brain, speech-language
    deficits in, 11
Legal and ethical considerations, 27
    advance directive planning, 123–124
    confidentiality, 36–37
    documentation, 38–39
    duty to protect third parties, 39
    electronic messaging systems and, 109
    email, 122–123
    information technology and security, 38
    professional boundaries, 39–41
    within Sunrise Model, 163
Leininger, Madeleine, 154, 163, 171, 173
Lifelong learning, 229, 230
Life span, culture and communication across,
    172–183
Life span considerations
    nurse–client relationships and, 113–119
    therapeutic communication techniques
        and, 84–90, 91
Linguistic biases, health care disparities and,
    160
Linguistic competence, 162
    defined, 154
Linguistics, 155
    defined, 154
Listening
    active, 57–59
    good, 58
    reflective, 79

M

Magnet designation, 205
Magnet Recognition Program, 205
Make-A-Wish Foundation, Web site for, 152
McKee, A., 200
Medical records
    confidentiality of, 123
    electronic, 38
    secure, 36

Medication adherence, assertiveness and
negotiation skills in, 68–69
Medscape/WebMD, Web site for, 152
Melnyk, B. M., 115
Mental health, self-renewal and, 229
Mentoring, 203
team-building skills through, 224
Middle adulthood
nurse–client relationship and, 117–118
therapeutic communication techniques
and, 88–89
Minorities
changing demographics and, 157
nurse–client relationship and, 19
Mistrust, 19

N

National Black Association for Speech-
Language and Hearing, Web site for, 97
National Guideline Clearinghouse, Web site
for, 152
National Hospice and Palliative Care
Organization, Web site for, 152
National Institute of Mental Health Outreach,
Web site for, 52
National Institute on Deafness and Other
Communication Disorders, Web sites for,
52, 97
Native American culture
humor within, 168
silence and, 167
NBASLH. *See* National Black Association for
Speech-Language and Hearing
Negotiation, 74–75, 91, 215
defined, 54, 196
skills, 215–217
Negotiation process, knowledge of, 216
Neurobiology, of language and
communication, 10–11
Neurodevelopmental disorders, 15
NIDCD. *See* National Institute on Deafness
and Other Communication Disorders
Nonfluent (or expressive) aphasia, 12
Nonverbal behaviors, meaning conveyed via,
33–34

Nonverbal communication, 5
assertiveness and, 63, 65
defined, 54
evaluating, 166
listening and, 58
professional assertiveness and, 206
Norming stage, in team development, 223,
224*t*
Núñez, A. E., 161
Nurse–client relationship, 103–107
challenges to integrity of, 101
cultural factors and, 18–19
defined, 100
empathy within, 30–31
exploitation phase in, 107
identification phase in, 106–107
impact of anxiety and stress on, 31–33
individualization of, 55–56
infancy and childhood and, 114–115
life span considerations in, 113–119
manner in which message is delivered in,
31
orientation phase in, 104–106
phases of, 6
psychosocial factors and, 18
rapport in, 28–29
resolution phase in, 107
self-awareness, personal development,
and, 111–113
telemedicine and, 26
trust in, 29–30
Nurse leaders, mentoring by, 203
Nurse–physician communication, disruptive
behaviors and, 4–5
Nurses
assertiveness and, 60
Code of Ethics for, 36
communication skills needed by, 4
cultural distinctions between clients and,
155
culturally competent, 164
death and dying issues, and self-awareness
in, 131, 140
essential characteristics in, 23*t*
health promotion for, 229
personal empowerment and, 197

as pivotal members of interdisciplinary
    teams, 222
stressful encounters and role of, 32–33
supportive relationships among, 203
transitions in health care and role of, 199
Nursing: Scope and Standards of Practice
    (ANA), 203
Nursing, within context of nurse–client
    relationship, 100
Nursing care, within Sunrise Model, 163
Nursing home decision, example dialogue,
    139–140
Nursing profession, culturally diverse, 158

O

Obsessive-compulsive disorder, 14
Office for Civil Rights, Web site for, 52
Office of Minority Health Information Center:
    Assuring Cultural Competence in Health
    Care, Web sites for, 238
Older adulthood
    communication during, 23–26
    culture and communication and,
        182–183
    nurse–client relationship and, 118–119
    therapeutic communication techniques
        and, 89
Older adults, major barriers to effective
    communication with, 24*t*
Online technologies, collaboration and, 123
Open-ended questions, 76–77
    example dialogue, 76–77
    terminal care and, 134
Opportunities, providing, effective leaders
    and, 202
Orientation phase
    example dialogue, 105–106
    in nurse–client relationship, 6, 104–106

P

Pagers, 4, 38
Palliative care, 124–125
Palm Pilots, 56

Parents. *See also* Children; Families
    dying or seriously ill child or adolescent
        and, 126
    nurse–client relationship with, 114–115
    therapeutic communication techniques
        and, 85–87
Park Ridge Center for Health, Faith, and
    Ethics, Web site for, 238
Passive communication, 60
    comparison of assertive communication,
        aggressive communication and, 61*t*
Passiveness, 65
Patient Self-Determination Act and Cruzan
    decision, 123–124, 137
Paulanka, B. J., 170
PBS Children's Hospital Parents Center, Web
    site for, 152
Peer pressure, during adolescence, 22, 87
Peplau, H. E., 6, 9, 103, 104, 107, 114
Peplau's interpersonal relations theory, 6–7
Perception, 14
Performance anxiety, 202
    public speaking and, 225
Performing stage, in team development, 223,
    224*t*
Personal ambitions, keeping in check, 201
Personal development, self-awareness and,
    111–113
Personal distance, 34, 170–171
Personal mastery, defined, 196
Personal space, 2
    nurse–client relationship and, 34–35
Physical health, self-renewal and, 229
Physician–nurse communication, disruptive
    behaviors and, 4–5
Piaget, J., 127
Politics, within Sunrise Model, 163
Polypharmacy, older adulthood and, 118
Positive attitude, negotiation and, 215
Positive treatment outcomes, communication
    and, 3
Praying, dying or seriously ill child or
    adolescent and, 127
Prejudice, evidence of, 210
Privacy, 27, 36
    electronic messaging systems and, 109

Professional assertiveness, 206–207
    essential characteristics of, 207t
Professional beliefs, within Sunrise Model,
    163
Professional boundaries, 2, 39–41
    strategies facilitating, 40t
Professional development, 204, 230
    leading through effective communication,
        195–230
Psychiatric conditions, personal space issues
    and, 35
Psychological health, self-renewal and, 229
Psychosocial issues, in communication, 15–18
Public distance, 34, 171
Public speaking skills, 225–227
    developing, 225–226
    major advantages of, 227
Purnell, L., 170

Q

Quality of health care, equitable health care
    and, 162
Quality time with patients, advocating for, 102
Questioning, 75–79
    closed-ended, 77–79
    defined, 54
    open-ended, 76–77

R

Race
    health care disparities and, 159–162, 165
    nurse–client relationship and, 19
Rapport, 2, 3, 55
    defined, 54
    effective communication and, 28–29
    orientation phase and, 104
    telemedicine and, 110
Reflection, 79–80
    defined, 54
    example dialogue, 79
Reflective listening, 79
    effective communication and, 202
Reimbursement for health care,
    documentation and, 39

Relationship management, effective leadership
    and, 200
Religion, within Sunrise Model, 163
Religious beliefs
    culture and, 156
    shared decision making and, 210
Religious practices, cultural sensitivity,
    families and, 180
Reporting laws, child abuse, elder abuse and,
    39
Resolution phase, in nurse–client relationship,
    6, 107
Right hemisphere of brain
    early secure attachments and, 20
    pivotal role of, in stress and coping
        responses, 16
Right to consent, 37
Robert Wood Johnson Publications and
    Resources, Web site for, 238
Rogers, Carl, 29
Roy, C., 103

S

Sahler, O. J., 128, 129
Satir, Virginia, 7, 8
Schiavo, Terry, 124
Schizophrenia, 12
    auditory hallucinations in, 14–15
    personal space issues and, 35
Secure attachments, cognitive component of,
    16
Secure attachments style, during infancy,
    20–21
Security, 123
    electronic messaging systems and, 109
    information technology and, 38
Self-awareness, 2, 17, 31, 101
    about space, 171
    cultural competence and, 165–166, 184
    cultural sensitivity and, 161–162
    death and dying issues and, 131, 140
    defined, 100
    earnest decision making and, 203–204
    effective leadership and, 200
    emotional intelligence and, 200

nonverbal cues and, 34
personal development and, 111–113
shared decision making and, 209
Self-concept, during adolescence, 87
Self-disclosure, 80–81
defined, 54
example dialogue, 80
Self-esteem, during adolescence, 87
Self-renewal
defined, 196
as forgotten leadership competence,
227–229
Self-worth, older adulthood and, 24
Sensory deficits, age-related, communication
difficulties and, 136–137
Sensory-perceptual influences, on
communication, 13–15
Sensory systems, 14
Sexual orientation, health care disparities and,
160
Shared decision making, 102, 122, 207–212
cultural and ethnic influences on,
209–212
culturally sensitive, facilitating, 212*t*
defined, 100
negotiation skills and, 215–217
women and, 177, 178
Silence
defined, 54
as therapeutic intervention, 81
Skopec, W. M., 215
Social awareness, effective leadership and, 200
Social distance, 34, 171
Social health, self-renewal and, 229
Social organization, cultural competence and,
172
Societal trends, in nurse–client relationships,
26
Socioeconomic status, health care disparities
and, 160
Space
cultural, 154
cultural competence and, 170–172
nurse–client relationship and, 34–35
Speakers, misperceptions contributing to
stifling of, 225

Speech, 2, 10
brain regions involved in, *11,* 11–12
disorders of, 12–13
infancy and development of, 21
Speech problems, early identification of, 22
Spiritual beliefs
culture and, 156
shared decision making and, 210
Spiritual health, self-renewal and, 229
Spirituality, within Sunrise Model, 163
Spiritual practices, cultural sensitivity, families
and, 180
Staff, therapeutic communication and, 56
Stage fright, 225
gaining control over, 226–227
Stakeholders, therapeutic communication and,
56
Stereotyping, 19, 118
health care disparities and, 160
self-awareness and recognition of, 112,
165
Storming stage, in team development, 223,
224*t*
Storytelling, by older adults, 24–25, 89,
118–119
Stress
impact of, on nurse–client relationship,
31–33
right hemisphere in brain and, 16
self-renewal and, 227–229
Strokes, 119
aphasias and, 12
depression and, 13
Stuttering, 12
Suicide risk, assessing for, in stroke patients,
13
Summarize technique, defined, 55
Summarizing, example dialogue, 82
Sunrise Model, 158
assessment process and, 173
concepts within, 163
Superior temporal gyrus, 11–12
Support systems, for older adults, 119
Sympathy, 2
empathy *vs.,* 30
Systems thinking, 205–206

T

Tarasoff v. Regents of University of California, 39
Team building, defined, 196
Team-building skills
    acquisition of, 217–224
        interdisciplinary teams, 220–224
Team development, stages of, 223
Team members, selection of, 221–222
Teams. *See also* Collaboration
    barriers associated with, 223
    developmental stages of, 224*t*
    ingredients for success of, 219*t*
    qualities in members of, 218
Technological and information systems, 26–27
Technology
    communication and, 4
    evidence-based care and, 198
    impact of, on interpersonal relations, 108–111
    within Sunrise Model, 163
Telehealth, 4
Telemedicine, 4, 26, 38, 110–111
    defined, 100
Terminally ill youth, communicating with, 130*t*
Text messages, 22
Therapeutic communication, 5
    benefits of, 55
    centrality of, to nursing, 90–91
    defined, 2, 55
    description of, 9–10
    key terms in, 2
    perspectives and principles of, 1–41
Therapeutic communication techniques, 53–91
    active listening, 57–59
    in adolescence, 87–88
    assertiveness, 59–61, 63–66
    clarification, 66–67
    conflict resolution, 67–69
    confrontation, 69–70
    family issues and, 85–87
    focusing, 71–72
    giving or imparting information, 72–73

    humor, 73
    in infancy and childhood, 84–85
    key terms for, 54–55
    life span considerations and, 84–90, 91
    in middle adulthood, 88–89
    negotiation, 74–75
    in older adulthood, 89
    questioning, 75–79
    reflection, 79–80
    self-disclosure, 80–81
    silence, 81
    summarizing, 82
    verbalizing the implied, 82–84
Third parties, duty to protect, 39
Time, cultural competence and, 168–170
Time out, 63
To Err is Human: Building a Safer Health System (Institute of Medicine), 197
Touch, importance of, during infancy, 114
Townsend, R., 201
Transactions, 2
    communication and, 3
    in experiential communication, 8
Transcultural care, 154
Tribal markings, 167
Tricultural interactions, health care system and, 161
Trust
    adolescence and, 23
    cultural awareness and, 19
    effective communication and, 29–30
    interdisciplinary teams and, 222
    nursing attributes and, 30
    orientation phase and, 104
    team-building and, 218
    telemedicine and, 110
Tuckerman, B., 221
Tulsky, J. A., 125

U

U.S. Census Bureau, 157
U.S. Department of Health and Human Services, Office of Minority Health, Web sites for, 193

V

Values, 155
    defined, 154
Verbal communication, 33
    evaluating, 166
    professional assertiveness and, 206
Verbalizing the implied, 82–84
    defined, 55
    example dialogue, 83
Video cameras, 56
Video recording, 4
Voice tone, effective communication and, 202
Von Gunten, G. F., 132

W

Web sites, security issues and, 109, 123
Wernicke's area, in brain, 2, 11, *11,* 12, 13, 14

Whalen v. United States, 123
Wisdom, effective leadership and, 204
Women, gender sensitivity considerations for, 177–180
Work-related stressors, 202
    identifying, 228
Work relationships, ANA definition of levels of, 221
Worldview, within Sunrise Model, 163

Y

Youth, terminally ill, communicating with, 130*t. See also* Adolescence